Dynamic Medicine

Dynamic Medicine

The World According to Homeopathy

Larry Malerba, D.O.

M

Maverick Press
New York

Dynamic Medicine
The World According to Homeopathy

Copyright © 2016 Larry Malerba
All rights reserved worldwide.

First Edition December, 2016
Maverick Press, Altamont, New York

Cover Art: Samuel Hahnemann Memorial, Washington, DC.
Source: Wikicommons, image in the public domain.

Typesetting and cover design: FormattingExperts.com

All quotations in this book are believed to be in accordance with Fair Use guidelines.

No portion of this book, except for brief quotations in reviews and educational articles, may be reproduced, stored, or transmitted in any form—digital, mechanical, photocopying, recording, or otherwise—without the prior written permission of the author.

For more information, contact Maverick Press: maverickpressbooks@gmail.com

Medical Disclaimer: All content in this book is intended for educational purposes only and should not be construed as medical advice or any other kind of professional advice for anyone reading these materials. This information is not intended as a substitute for consultation with a qualified health care professional. All readers are encouraged to seek appropriate counsel in the event of a health problem.

ISBN: 978-0-9980134-0-4

Contents

Foreword xi

CHAPTER 1. Beginnings 1

CHAPTER 2. Who Seeks Homeopathic Care and Why? 17

CHAPTER 3. Some Homeopathic Case Histories 25

CHAPTER 4. Remedies and References 49

CHAPTER 5. How to Explain Homeopathy? Let Me Count the Ways.... 63

CHAPTER 6. How We Get Sick and Why 89

CHAPTER 7. Homeopathic Psychology 123

CHAPTER 8. The True Nature of Health and Healing 143

CHAPTER 9. Common Misconceptions 169

CHAPTER 10. The Revolutionary Nature of Homeopathic Healing . . . 191

Appendix of Practical Homeopathic Tips 221

Epigraphs & Notes 233

About the Author 249

*This book is dedicated to all those warriors, past and present,
who have fought for truth and labored out of love for homeopathy*

Acknowledgments

- I could not have accomplished this project without the unyielding support of my beautiful wife, Mary, who served as advisor, editor, critic, and cheerleader all rolled into one.
- Special thanks to Francis Treuherz for his support. His deep knowledge of the homeopathic literature is truly inspiring.
- Many thanks to the Formatting Experts for their publishing advice and technical assistance.

Foreword

Francis Treuherz, MA RSHom FSHom

> *I have often had physicians tell me that it was due to suggestion that my medicines acted so well; but my answer to this is, that I suggest just as strongly with my wrong remedy as with the right one, and my patients improve only when they have received the similar or correct remedy.*
>
> –James Tyler Kent, MD (1926)

Larry Malerba has written a book that I wish I had written. I cannot pay him a higher compliment than this. He has illuminated the mindset of homeopaths, which will help the gentle reader understand how we think. At the same time, writing from his considerable training and experience, he has been able to compare homeopathic thinking with conventional thinking. The result will help new patients and student homeopaths alike understand what we are about, and what they will be pleased to leave behind. Experienced colleagues will find that their ideas are expanded, clarified and reinforced. This is a book for everyone.

I was a successful patient over 40 years ago and there was no work like this to help me overcome the mysteries of homeopathy, just my Clarke's *Dictionary*,[i] until I discovered Kent's *Philosophy*,[ii] which of course reminded me of Clark Kent. Then I found my trusted Boericke's *Pocket Manual*,[iii] which I read on the subway and people thought it was a Bible. They were correct. Since then I have trained and become a homeopath, and my wife says that now I have two religions.

But joking apart, homeopathy is not a religion, although it can become a way of life. The author explains that belief is not necessary for therapeutic success. It works on animals that have no conception of placebo, and it works on sceptical academic physicists who appear as patients when their wives insist. I had one such patient who would not come back to see me when the homeopathic medicine was effective—his wife reported he was too embarrassed. My response to the sceptics would be to invite them to participate in a blinded proving of the remedy *Aesculus hippocastanum*, and let them suffer the consequences.*

Remedy pictures and patient stories are presented in a readable yet serious style. The author's tale of prescribing for his mother is very moving and echoes my own experience, which I documented in 'My Son the Homeopath.' Larry Malerba has written what I hope will become a modern classic. I have learned from it, and confirmed much that I already knew, from the fresh, erudite and entertaining way he has presented the ideas of empirical versus rational medicine in counterpoint.

---

i. John Henry Clarke, *Dictionary of Practical Materia Medica* in 3 volumes, Homœopathic Publishing Company, London, 1900-1902.

ii. James Tyler Kent, *Lectures on Homeopathic Philosophy*, Ehrhart & Karl, Chicago, 1900.

iii. William Boericke & Oscar Boericke, *Pocket Manual of Homeopathic Materia Medica comprising the Characteristic and Guiding Symptoms of the Remedies, with a Repertory*, Boericke & Runyon, Philadelphia, 9th edition, 1927.

* In a proving, test subjects take repeated doses of a homeopathic remedy in order to study the symptoms that it can cause, and the symptoms that it can therefore treat. *Aesculus hippocastanum* produces the following very uncomfortable symptoms: 'Rectum: dry, aching. Feels full of small sticks. Anus raw, sore. Much pain after stool, with prolapse. Haemorrhoids; with sharp shooting pains up the back; blind and bleeding.' (Boericke 1927).

CHAPTER 1
Beginnings

> *It is not so that our first duty is to our patient. Our first duty is to the truth, which, when loyally served, best enables us to do the greatest good to the sick.*
> –E. A. Farrington, MD (1936)

> *It has often been said that homeopathy existed before Hahnemann. So it did; in the same way as gravity existed before Newton.*
> –Margery Blackie, MD,
> Physician to Her Majesty, the Queen (1976)

Homeopathic healing is a truly powerful and mysterious phenomenon. The capacity for homeopathy to heal the whole person is unparalleled. No other system of healing shatters the illusion of separation of mind and body so completely. It also happens to be one of the most controversial and hotly debated topics on the planet today. By one measure, *Homeopathy* is the second most highly contested page on *Wikipedia*, runner-up only to the *Jesus* page.[1]

The crux of the matter centers on claims that it is not possible for tiny homeopathic doses of medicines to achieve the dramatic results that they achieve. On one side of the argument, skeptics and scientists demand an explanation that is compatible with their materialist conception of the natural world. On the other side, everyone from practitioners, to patients, to theoretical physicists propose a variety of tantalizing theories that, if taken seriously, could revolutionize the way we understand health and healing. The controversy over homeopathy rages on more feverishly than ever.

But I gave up long ago wondering *why* homeopathy works, and contented myself instead with knowing from experience that it *does* work. There is just no satisfactory way to explain the results that I have seen from treating thousands of patients—their acute and chronic physical, emotional, and mental illnesses—over the course of my long career.

Most people just don't get homeopathy until they experience it firsthand. It sounds too good to be true, and understandably so. For some, it can require a type of religious conversion, not in the sense of surrendering one's judgment to blind faith, but in the sense that one suddenly sees things from a different perspective. Such changes of perspective often come in the form of epiphanies that bring about a paradigm shift in thinking. And those changes of mind are usually prompted by unusual personal experiences. Overall restoration of personal health and well-being of mind and body is just the type of experience that homeopathic treatment can produce.

I was a teenage allopath

I grew up in a rather conventional, allopathically oriented environment. A good number of my parents' friends were doctors. My father's father was a doctor. My best friend's father was a doctor. My father made a point of instructing me to address his doctor friends respectfully, as "doctor" so and so. I remember being irked each time I heard my parents recommend a doctor to a friend. Their endorsement would always be accompanied by the standard qualifier that "he is the best in his field." I would think to myself, how can every doctor that they know be the best at what they do? Needless to say, people of that generation were inclined to revere doctors in a way that seemed a little too naïve to me.

Although my parents weren't exactly pill poppers, drugs and surgeries were viewed as routine aspects of life. I do remember one brief brush with pseudo-holism when I visited a pediatrician seeking help for warts on my knees. After acknowledging that he had nothing substantive to offer, the pediatrician told me to walk backwards around a flagpole thirteen times while reciting an incantation that I cannot now recall. I came away amused but unimpressed. I tried using *Compound W* for a while, but the warts remained. They eventually went away on their own—I'm not sure why.

My family wasn't particularly health-oriented. A number of relatives were alcoholics. And many were smokers. My mother was a chain smoker. It was nothing unusual for the time. Women smokers were "liberated" and cocktail parties were signs of sophistication. In retrospect, I don't know why, but I was not willing to accept convention.

Perhaps it had something to do with the time I asked my mother if I could smoke cigarettes. I was only a kid, but she agreed, under one condition. If I could light a cigarette and smoke the whole thing through to the end, then she would allow me to smoke. I took her up on her challenge. I don't think I got past three puffs before I was coughing, hacking, nauseous, and miserable. Talk about homeopathic parenting! She had allowed me to partake of the poison in order to cure me of the desire. Needless to say, I showed no interest in smoking cigarettes ever again.

As the years went by, I would orchestrate anti-smoking terror campaigns with the help of my siblings. I wasn't driven by any particular holistic belief; I just knew smoking wasn't good for my mother. We would steal, hide, and destroy her cigarettes. When that failed, we would argue with her, trying to coax and shame her into kicking the habit ... all to no avail.

I was very close to my mom's father who lived nearby. "Pop" was also a lifelong heavy smoker. As they grew older, I became the all-purpose caretaker of my grandparent's home and property. I was in high school when Pop was diagnosed with lung cancer. My family was not one to talk about issues, problems, or emotions. Pop was hospitalized, had an entire lung removed, and I guess it was just expected that he would recover and return home. I have a very sharp memory of visiting him after surgery. As I walked him gingerly up and down the hospital hallway, he eagerly stopped to introduce the nurses to his grandson. I beamed with pride.

While getting ready for school the next morning, the phone rang. I picked it up. When the voice on the other end said that it was the hospital calling, it was like a bolt of lightning. I honestly don't think I had seen it coming. I, too, had just assumed that medicine would save the day.

Fast forward thirty-plus years later and my mother was diagnosed with lung cancer. By then, I was a practicing homeopathic physician and she was still very much enamored of her conventional doctors. They told her it was a tiny spot that would only require the removal of a small portion of a lung. This time I wasn't fooled. I knew that she wasn't in good enough condition to undergo such a powerfully stressful experience. At the time, she was taking what seemed like a mile-long list of prescription drugs. She underwent surgery and then chemotherapy, during which time she was unquestionably debilitated for months on end. It took all her strength to simply sit in a recliner during her waking hours. Given so much allopathic drugging, I didn't think that homeopathy could be of much use. But one day, out of desperation, I asked her if she wanted my help anyway. She agreed to give it a try.

I sat down to take her case, asking her as many questions as I could when she wasn't nodding off to sleep. Her main complaint at the time was a combination of terrible nausea and weakness. While I believed that the nausea was a residual effect from the chemotherapy, it also dawned on me that my mother had spent a lifetime smoking like a chimney. I put two and two together and decided that *Tabacum*, the homeopathic remedy made from tobacco, might be a good choice. Homeopathic *Tabacum* is known to be useful in debilitating cases of nausea precisely because, in its crude form, it is capable of causing nausea and weakness. I instructed her to take two doses of *Tabacum* 30c.

I received a phone call from my sister two days later. She wanted to know what the heck I had given our mother. Now my sister had been our mother's regular caretaker, so she had grown accustomed to her chronic state of lethargy. But when she arrived at our mother's home that morning, she found her up and vacuuming the carpets. She was dumbstruck because for months our mother hadn't gotten up from her chair for any other reason than to use the bathroom. Suddenly, there she was cleaning the house!

Fortunately, *Tabacum* seemed to do the job. She continued to do well and never fell back into that debilitating state of nausea. My mother survived a few more years under constant allopathic care before she ultimately succumbed. I suspect that without the *Tabacum*, she would not have lasted even that long. In contrast to my Pop's death, I was profoundly aware of the circumstances that had preceded my mother's death.

So what is homeopathy anyway?

I remember back in medical school when I first encountered the exotic sounding names of homeopathic medicines: *Ferrum phosphoricum, Crotalus horridus, Aconitum napellus,* and many more. A strange new world opened up before me as I paged through my homeopathic reference books. Dr. Kirby Hotchner had recommended the books to his class. Dr. Hotchner was a professor of family practice medicine who was somehow permitted to teach an elective homeopathy course in an allopathic medical school. The whole thing became a little less mysterious when I realized that those remedy names were written in Latin. They were the genus and species of plants and animals and the Latin identifiers of elements and minerals. What had previously seemed like some ancient indecipherable language, now took on a more scientific flavor. Of course, it's all second nature to me now. Homeopathy has become the lens through which I view life, health, illness, and healing. And, yes, homeopathy can have that kind of effect on a person.

As told in my first book, *Green Medicine*, it wasn't until after I graduated from osteopathic medical school, and after I had begun a solo practice in classical homeopathy, that I was told about an unusual detail regarding my family history. My good friend Chris Ellithorp, a talented homeopathic historian and archivist, was looking through an old directory of physicians one day when he discovered that my father's father had graduated in 1928 from New York Homeopathic Medical

College. As far as I can tell, he went on to practice conventional family medicine, dedicating much of his time to treating the poor. The topic never came up in my interactions with him when I was a teenager. Back then, I had never even heard of homeopathy. But somehow, the homeopathic influence had been passed on down to me.

This book is my attempt to convey to you, the reader, an understanding of the world as seen from a homeopathic perspective. My intention is to help you wrap your mind around the science, art, and mystery that is homeopathy. And believe me, while homeopathic methodology is indisputably scientific, and its practice requires an artful touch, the explanation for its remarkable power to heal remains a mystery, even to those who have successfully used it for many years.

Given the unusual nature of the subject, most homeopathy books begin with an obligatory explanation of this paradoxical system of healing. I will do the same, beginning here with a simple description. As we progress through the book I will explore some of the complexities and nuances of homeopathy, including the implications that it raises regarding the nature of life and human health and illness. So buckle up, here we go.

Since the topic tends to create a lot of confusion, it is important to begin with a statement regarding what homeopathy is not. It is not herbal medicine. Neither is it nutritional medicine. People commonly make the mistake of thinking that homeopathy and holistic medicine are the same thing. They are not. Holistic medicine is a broader term that includes a wide array of holistic therapies, like acupuncture, massage, herbal medicine, Traditional Chinese Medicine, and homeopathy. Homeopathy is a specific system of healing that can be categorized under the general heading of holistic medicine. Simply put, homeopathic medicine is a subset of holistic medicine.

The central tenet of homeopathy is very simple: the administration of small doses of a substance known to be able to cause symptoms similar to the symptom pattern of a sick individual can be used to treat that person and his or her illness. One could say that it is a "hair of the dog" approach to healing. The actual practice of homeopathy, however, is quite a bit more complex than that.

Just a little over two hundred years ago, a German physician, Dr. Samuel Hahnemann, serendipitously conceived of his revolutionary idea while translating a medical text that included a discussion of malaria. The book described the symptoms of malaria, referenced a type of tree bark (Cinchona) used to treat malaria, and then attributed the therapeutic action of the bark to its bitter taste and ability to disorder the stomach. Hahnemann being no fool was not impressed by this explanation and decided to investigate on his own.

Although he did not have malaria, Hahnemann nevertheless ingested doses of Cinchona bark in order to observe its effect. To his surprise, he developed symptoms typical of intermittent fever, a type of fever that can be easily mistaken for malaria. He surmised that Cinchona was a useful treatment for malaria because of the close resemblance between the symptoms that the bark caused and the actual symptoms of malaria. With this idea in mind, Hahnemann experimented with other substances, using himself and his family members as test subjects. These experiments with medicinal substances were the first of what Hahnemann later called his "provings." According to some, Hahnemann's provings are believed to be the first systematic drug trials in the annals of Western medicine.

Hahnemann studied the symptom profiles of a variety of substances and then prescribed them for individuals who reported having similar clusters of symptoms. He refined his method by reducing the doses of medicines given in the hope of avoiding toxic side effects. In doing so, Hahnemann noticed something rather peculiar. The lower doses seemed to have a more beneficial therapeutic effect. He diluted his medicines even further and was pleased to discover that they still worked. In this manner he was able to completely eliminate any potential toxicity.

By modern pharmacological standards, Hahnemann's medicines were so dilute as to be unable to cause any harm. And here is where the great controversy arises. In spite of their high degree of dilution, homeopathic medicines are not just placebos. They have an obvious ability to affect biological systems and they retain their capacity to heal a wide range of illnesses. This basic truth has been verified over and over again by homeopathic practitioners and their patients for the past two centuries. A growing body of scientific research indicates the same.

For example, it was Hahnemann himself who introduced ipecac into medical usage. Contemporary doctors know of ipecac's ability to produce nausea and vomiting. It is still used in emergency departments to induce vomiting to empty the stomach contents of individuals who have ingested suspected poisons or overdosed on drugs. Hahnemann, however, used ipecac for entirely different reasons. When a patient presented to him complaining of nausea and vomiting, he knew that homeopathically diluted doses of ipecac could be used to relieve those symptoms.

Dr. Hahnemann developed a standardized process by which to make his medicines. He would dilute the original crude substance in some kind of solvent and then shake it vigorously. One part of the resulting solution was then placed in more solvent, thereby diluting it further. The new solution was then succussed—or shaken—again. This process of *serial dilution and succussion* was repeated a specified number of times until the desired potency was obtained. The numbers and letters that follow the names of homeopathic medicines are notations that indicate the degree of serial dilution and succussion. (For example: 3x, 30c, 200x, 1M, and so on) Hahnemann called this process by which he transformed crude substances into their corresponding homeopathic remedies *potentization*.

After potentizing his medicines in order to remove their gross toxicity, Hahnemann was amazed to find that they were, nevertheless, capable of producing a more global effect than he had anticipated. Since it was not possible that such highly diluted medicines could act in a manner similar to material doses of conventional drugs, Hahnemann shrewdly theorized that they must act on some immaterial plane in some mysterious energetic fashion. Based upon their clinical observations, Hahnemann and his successors knew that homeopathic medicines were not chemical medicines; they were much more. Ernest A. Farrington, MD, an 1868 graduate of the Hahnemann Medical College of Philadelphia, understood that as a homeopathic physician he was "dealing with forces" that defied conventional scientific explanation.

> *Hahnemann did not belong to the materialistic school. To him the plant or root from which he made his tincture was not inert matter alone, but contained a living principle which was not nature but life. He knew that he was dealing with forces which transcended his natural senses, except in so far as their activities were displayed in their workings through matter. Hence his studies led him to the process of potentization of drugs. ... his remedies were free to act above the crude laws of physics, independent of gravity and of chemistry, but still within the bounds of matter.*[2]

If it was true that Hahnemann's remedies were too dilute to have a crude pharmacological effect, and if it was true that they exerted their influence on an as-of-yet undetectable dynamic energetic plane, then it must be the case that they interact with a similar underlying dynamic energy that presumably organizes and directs the homeostatic activities of the human organism.

Hahnemann documented the principles of his new system of medicine in 1810 in the 1st edition of his groundbreaking *Organon*.[3] Here, in a translation of the final 6th edition from the original German, Hahnemann defines the governing principle that animates all living beings. He alternately referred to it in his writings as *dynamis*, the *life force*, and the *vital force*.

> *In the healthy human state, the spirit-like life force that enlivens the material organism as dynamis, governs without restriction and keeps all parts of the organism in admirable, harmonious, vital operation, as regards both feelings and functions, so that our indwelling, rational spirit can freely avail itself of this living, healthy instrument for the higher purposes of our existence.*[4]

Hahnemann's genius was that he built a practical system of therapeutics capable of transcending crude pharmacological medicine. The spirit essence of the correctly chosen medicine, one that matches the symptom profile of the suffering patient, resonates with the spiritual dynamis of the organism—the life force—and acts upon it in such a way as to bring about restoration of health. Here, in his own words, Hahnemann grasps the true power of his discovery:

> *The smallest dose of a medicine dynamized in the best manner gives out, in the appropriate disease case, more curative energy by far than large doses of the same medicinal substance.*[5]

If, as Hahnemann believed, all illness springs from an out-of-balance life force, then no strictly chemical or biological intervention is capable setting it straight. Illness that develops from the dynamic interplay of energetic forces requires a similarly dynamic therapeutic agent to restore balance to the life force.

> *Our life force, as spirit-like dynamis, cannot be seized and affected by damaging impingements on the healthy organism other than in a spirit-like, dynamic way. ... Accordingly, curative medicines can reestablish health and life's harmony only through dynamic action on the life principle.*[6]

Hahnemann believed that this strange and paradoxical dose-dependent phenomenon was a virtual law of nature. Not surprisingly, he called it the "law of similars." Any substance known to be able to generate a certain set of symptoms in its crude form should, therefore, be able to be used in diluted homeopathic form to treat similar symptoms. It was upon the foundation of this bedrock principle that Dr. Hahnemann built his renowned system of healing.

Technically speaking, it was not Hahnemann's discovery. Paracelsus, Hippocrates, and others had contemplated the idea before him. Hahnemann did manage, however, to devise a practical means by which to put the idea into action. Amazingly, as Hahnemann would soon discover, his new method was capable of treating not just physical illness, but also emotional disorders and mental illness as well.

It is important to realize that although Hahnemann used symptoms as *clues* to determine the course of treatment, symptoms were *not the object* of treatment. He sought to accomplish much more than that. His intent was not just to treat symptoms as much as the person experiencing those symptoms. To his great delight, Hahnemann discovered that treatment based on the paradoxical principle of similars was capable of doing just that.

Hahnemann's diluted medicines didn't just bring temporary relief from specific symptoms. He repeatedly observed that the correct remedy, or *simillimum*, could relieve his patients' symptoms permanently while at the same time restoring their overall health and well-being. In other words, homeopathic remedies seemed to act in a manner completely different from conventional drugs. While most drugs provide only temporary symptomatic relief, homeopathic medicines could be used to rebuild the health of a sick person. The implications of his discovery were truly profound, indeed.

Allow me to illustrate the paradox of homeopathic healing with a couple of concrete examples. Contact with the poison ivy plant can result in a familiar set of symptoms that we would all rather avoid. Those same symptoms provide the guide for the proper use of the homeopathically diluted version of poison ivy, which is known as *Rhus toxicodendron* (*Rhus tox* in shortened form). Now, there happen to be other medical conditions that can exhibit symptom patterns similar to poison ivy. Think for a moment about the similarity between poison ivy and chicken pox, for example. Now consider herpes, shingles, and even some cases of dermatitis. All of these conditions can manifest similarly with itching, blistering, and oozing discharges. Most homeopathic practitioners are aware of this similarity and have used *Rhus tox* at one time or another to successfully treat all of these conditions.

Think now about the pattern of symptoms associated with the honeybee. The typical redness, swelling, pain, and itching caused by a bee sting should come to mind. Now consider other health problems that can manifest in a similar manner. How about hives, allergy symptoms, or an allergic reaction? Redness, swelling, and itching are symptoms common to all three. Even some sore throats can manifest as redness, swelling, and pain. In all such conditions, *Apis mellifica*, the homeopathic remedy made from the honeybee, can be very helpful, especially when the symptoms of the condition closely match the symptoms of the remedy.

Let's try another example. Jimson Weed, also known as *Datura stramonium*, is a plant from the nightshade family. It grows in the wild and has flowers that bloom at night. The plant is poisonous and can induce a variety of very unpleasant symptoms including paranoia, restlessness, agitation, and terrifying hallucinations. In homeopathic usage it is referred to as *Stramonium*. Homeopaths have studied the symptom profile of *Stramonium* in great detail. It produces a spectrum of symptoms that fit the general idea of fight or flight. One end of the spectrum includes irritability, anger, aggression, and rage, while the other manifests as anxiety, paranoia, and certain specific fears. Those fears include fear of the dark, water, animals, and fear of being alone, especially at night.

Not surprisingly, homeopaths have found *Stramonium* to be a very useful medicine in cases that exhibit a similar fight or flight pattern of symptoms. Victims of physical trauma and sexual abuse often fit the profile. War veterans with PTSD and children with ADHD can also exhibit similar symptoms. Perhaps one of the more common uses of homeopathic *Stramonium* is for children with night terrors who are afraid of the dark and afraid to sleep alone at night. As you can see, homeopathic medicines are used to treat psychological problems as well as physical ones.

Individualization of care is the final piece to the homeopathic puzzle. Homeopaths understand that all cases of illness are unique—even when the conventional diagnosis is the same. Each person's illness must be met on its own terms. For example, not all cases of PTSD are the same. It cannot be said that Stramonium is *the* indicated remedy for PTSD. Ten cases of PTSD may require ten different homeopathic medicines. The thing that makes one particular case of PTSD different from all other cases of PTSD may be the very factor that determines the choice of homeopathic remedy. Distinguished author, Wilhelm Ameke, MD, underscores the point that Dr. Hahnemann was a pioneer who stressed the importance of individualized treatment as a cornerstone of homeopathic care.

> *Hahnemann deserves the credit of having insisted upon the strictest individualization of diseases, and he showed its necessity more conclusively than any other physician. Classification is so convenient and easy that most medical men incline to it. Hahnemann always advocated individualization, and taught it systematically in his numerous works.*[7]

The homeopathic answer to a great deal of human suffering has been hiding in plain sight for over two hundred years now. The odd thing is that when people are told of this not-so-secret secret, many show little interest. I suspect that this is because they are confident that, when the time comes, conventional medicine will provide for their needs. They have been conditioned by the media, by the educational system, and by conventional medical culture to believe that science already provides the best healthcare that there is to be had. Such is the bane of any homeopathic practitioner's existence. We know there is a better way, but only a few are interested in learning more about it.

Questions invariably arise, however, when conventional medicine lets people down, which it often does. People's illusions regarding the competence of the medical system can be shattered when the side effects of treatment become intolerable or when relief from their illnesses eludes them. Unfortunately, many tend to seek alternative care late in the game, after their conditions have had months or even years to progress. In spite of the fact that the average homeopathic doctor treats a large number of such late-stage cases, the outcomes can be remarkably positive.

This book is my attempt to provide an insider's understanding of what homeopathy is all about. Included herein are a number of case histories, a variety of hypotheses regarding the mysterious mechanism behind homeopathy, an explanation for the real reasons why people become ill, a comparison of the differences between suppressive allopathic treatment and genuine homeopathic healing, insight into the homeopathic perspective regarding psychology and mind-body phenomena, a discussion of homeopathic politics, and a great deal more. If you are unfamiliar with homeopathy, this book should turn your understanding of the nature of health, illness, and healing on its head. Even if you are already familiar with the topic, I hope it will still give you much food for thought.

The fact is that homeopathy has the power to heal medical conditions that orthodox medicine has little to offer. It is also true that the way in which homeopathy does that is a complete mystery. For this reason, it is a topic of great controversy, one that has its defenders and its detractors. I have always believed that the lack of scientific explanation for homeopathy is essentially irrelevant. To ponder over why homeopathy works is a peripheral issue, a luxury for philosophers and scientists to debate. All that really matters is whether or not it works. As far as I am concerned, there is no doubt as to the answer to that question.

This book represents my own personal take on homeopathy. Many familiar with the topic will agree with me; some will disagree. That is as it should be. After all, homeopathy is both art and science. Homeopathy is both a science and an experience-based discipline that has much to teach to patient and practitioner. Those experiences form the foundation of our ever-evolving understanding of health, illness, and healing.

Homeopathy is a collaborative undertaking, the lessons of which often clash with the conventional paternalistic medical understanding of the way things work. Since the conventional medical perspective is our default medical perspective, it will be necessary to frequently compare and contrast the two systems. Homeopathy does not invalidate orthodox medicine as much as it provides a fresh perspective on human health and healing.

In the final analysis, I believe that the best of all medical worlds—homeopathic, allopathic, and all other holistic systems—must be synergistically combined in order to minister effectively to the sick and the suffering. With that said, oftentimes the best and most effective first line of defense is homeopathy.

About footnotes: You will notice that in addition to their normal usage, I have placed footnotes in certain locations where I describe particular health problems or sets of symptoms. The idea is to create a fun exercise for those who wish to guess what homeopathic remedy might be indicated for the situation. Most cases involve actual patients and the actual remedies given. Others represent hypothetical situations. Naturally, this is for the benefit of those with some knowledge of homeopathy. However, it is not intended to, and should by no means deter newcomers to homeopathy from reading this book.

About terminology: I make frequent references to *conventional medicine* throughout the book. So as not to be repetitive, I also use similar terms including *orthodox medicine*, *mainstream medicine*, *Western medicine*, and *allopathic medicine*. For my purposes here, they are all used to refer to the same thing: conventional medicine. Likewise, I use the terms *life force* and *vital force* interchangeably. The same applies to my use of the terms, *homeopathic remedies* and *homeopathic medicines*. When the word *drug* or *medicine* comes up on its own, without the *homeopathic* qualifier, it is usually a reference to conventional pharmaceutical drugs. When *remedy* appears alone it indicates a homeopathic medicine.

CHAPTER 2

Who Seeks Homeopathic Care and Why?

> *Although it has spread to all parts of the civilized world, numbering its practitioners by thousands and its patients by millions, homeopathy has never found open and general acceptance in the medical profession. ... It is only another illustration of the fact that poets, prophets, and philosophers often perceive great truths and announce them to the world long before slow-moving scientists succeed in proving them to their own satisfaction.*
> –Stuart Close, MD (1924)

Is there a typical homeopathic patient?

Although the type of person who seeks homeopathic treatment varies according to region, culture, and the reputation and expertise of the individual practitioner, it is also generally true that women are more inclined to give homeopathy a try. As a rule, they are more open to holistic healing methods compared to men who are often more skeptical of anything that does not meet with mainstream scientific approval. Of course, I do not mean to say that all men and women fit the stereotype. There are plenty of exceptions.

The scenario usually unfolds along these lines: A mother schedules an appointment to consult with me about her own health issues. She meets with success in treating those problems and finds homeopathy to her liking, largely because it is safe, effective, unlikely to produce side effects, and allows her to rely less on pharmaceutical drugs. Soon thereafter, she brings her children in for treatment.

Only well after the family has established a successful treatment record does the husband reluctantly schedule an appointment. He usually begins the consultation with a qualifying statement that goes something like this: "My wife wanted me to see you. I don't believe in this stuff, but I'll give it a try." If I'm lucky enough to choose an effective remedy on the first try, then I may have a convert on my hands. If not, it is unlikely that I will see dad again. Again, this is not to say that there aren't plenty of men who are receptive to homeopathy in spite of its unconventional status. Not surprisingly, the clientele of many homeopathic practices consist mainly of women and children.

It should be noted that in its heyday back in the 1800s, homeopathy became popular partly due to its accessibility. First aid remedy kits and first aid homeopathy books were common items in the household. Since the typical home was many miles from the nearest physician, homeopathic or otherwise, it fell to the woman of the house to learn the art of first aid prescribing for family members. If you are at all familiar with the healing power of homeopathy, you know how valuable that must have been in the absence of a local doctor. The historic role of women in the early growth of homeopathy should not be underestimated.

Many choose homeopathy because they have become disillusioned with orthodox medical care. They have experienced firsthand the shortcomings of the medical system. They have gone the rounds, tried all that medicine has to offer, and still find themselves struggling with health issues that have not abated. They do the research looking for alternatives, discover homeopathy, and decide to give it a try. Most homeopathic practices are filled with patients whose ailments have not responded to conventional medical care. In this very real sense, homeopathic practitioners are often faced with the most difficult cases, the ones that regular doctors have become frustrated with because they have nothing more to offer.

Of course, there are also those who choose homeopathic care simply because it is compatible with their general philosophy of health. Contrary to the stereotype of holistic health care consumers as granolas, hippies, New Agers, or what have you, they tend to be well-educated, health-conscious individuals who are concerned about the dangers of conventional drugs and prefer a safer and more natural approach. They represent a large subculture within society whose understanding of health, illness, and its treatment is not often reflected in mainstream culture.

It is undeniable that there is a growing cultural divide between those who place their trust in the medical system and those who reluctantly resort to conventional care only when necessary. The latter tend to rely on a variety of legitimate holistic options at their disposal. The schism is unfortunate; it doesn't have to be this way. Notwithstanding the fact that the divide is largely a function of closed-mindedness on the part of the medical establishment, I still advise my patients that it is best to maintain good relationships with their regular doctors in the event that they may someday need their services.

A key factor that creates resistance to homeopathy in the United States is the fact that homeopathic medicines cannot be patented. For this reason, PhRMA (Pharmaceutical Research and Manufacturers of America) has no interest in homeopathy. It represents small potatoes compared to the earning power of blockbuster drugs. On the other hand, it poses a threat to Big Medicine's mainstream monopoly on health care. Those who regularly use homeopathy tend to be less dependent upon conventional medical services. A remedy kit with one hundred different medicines, for example, can be purchased from a homeopathic supplier for less than a couple hundred dollars. Such a kit can serve a family's first aid medical needs for many years. For this reason, homeopathy is ideal for poor nations where medical care is sparse and unaffordable for most. Homeopathy is the safest, least expensive, and most effective option available to third world countries. Ironically, homeopathic services must often be paid for out-of-pocket in the U.S. since it is not covered by most insurance policies.

Lastly, homeopathy requires that patients be willing to forego the instant gratification, pill-popping lifestyle embraced by so many. Homeopathy discourages the routine practice of symptom suppression and encourages patience when it comes to the treatment of illness. Once a homeopathic medicine is prescribed, a patient may be asked to wait for a period of weeks or even months before taking any additional homeopathic remedies.

Homeopathic practitioners understand that it is counterproductive to treat most symptoms without taking into account the larger context. Homeopathic care requires a longer view, one that measures success by the long-term results, not the day-to-day fluctuations of individual symptoms. This is not to say that homeopathy takes longer to work than conventional drugs. In fact, when a correct medicine is administered, it often works quite rapidly.

Why do patients seek homeopathic care?

The answer to this question is pretty straightforward. People seek homeopathic treatment for all kinds of reasons. They use homeopathy for physical, emotional, and mental health problems in all stages, acute and chronic. These are the people who know about homeopathy. The problem, however, is that most people have little awareness of homeopathy and even less knowledge regarding the types of problems that it can help.

I suspect that most practitioners would agree with me when I say that it is difficult to have to sit back and watch people suffer needlessly. This is because, from my perspective, although help is available, most people are unaware of it. I have also found from experience that most people don't believe it when I tell them that homeopathy can be effective for their particular health issue. They just assume that I mean well but that homeopathy is no different from all the herbs and nutritionals that line the shelves in the typical natural health store. I have found this to be true even of friends and relatives.

Years ago, I was puzzled by the matter-of-fact responses from some when I suggested that homeopathy might be a beneficial avenue to explore. I grew frustrated, for example, by the lack of interest on the part of a friend who repeatedly complained about his child's behavior problems. Each time he brought up the topic, I explained to him that homeopathy can help such problems—to no avail.

With time I learned that it is not my place to convince people of the virtues of homeopathy. I came to realize that it is only possible to reach those who are receptive. It is human nature to resist when being coaxed or pressured into doing something that one feels unsure about. Trying to persuade someone who is not receptive can be a counterproductive use of one's energy. It can be painful to keep one's thoughts to oneself in such instances, knowing that help will not be accepted even when that help can make a positive difference.

For those willing to try, homeopathy can be a game changer. It completely alters the playing field upon which the art and science of medicine is conducted. Conventional medicine limits itself to the physical manifestations of illness. This accounts for why it has so much trouble handling complex problems that have their origins in the psyche. The homeopathic playing field is far broader. It encompasses all that can be discerned on physical, emotional, mental, and spiritual levels.

Furthermore, orthodox medical treatment is handicapped by a rigid set of preformulated diagnostic categories. Those diagnoses constitute the foundation of one-size-fits-all, cookie-cutter medicine. Persons whose ailments do not meet such criteria are fated to be shuffled from specialist to specialist, who can be tempted to impose ill-suited diagnostic labels even when they are not warranted. Homeopathy bypasses the need for this type of stereotyping and focuses instead on the specific complaints of each individual patient. Although diagnostic information can be helpful in understanding the nature of a health problem, it is not always necessary for successful homeopathic prescribing.

The good news is that homeopathy has no problem with all those misfit patients who fall between the diagnostic cracks of conventional medicine. It does not get bogged down or distracted by the diagnostic name game. Diagnostic labels are really just convenient allopathic caricatures of the diverse symptom profiles of actual patients. Such diagnoses are too general and not specific enough for the purposes of homeopathic prescribing.

It is not sufficient to know, for example, that a patient has been given a diagnosis of pneumonia. A homeopath must understand the patient's symptoms in much greater detail in order to successfully treat that specific case of pneumonia. One patient with pneumonia may describe a dry cough that becomes worse with any movement. X-rays reveal that the pneumonia is confined to the right lung. (Remedy choice?[8]) Another person reports a cough that makes a rattling sound, as if the chest is filled with mucus. Nevertheless, all efforts to cough up the mucus fail. (Remedy choice?[9]) The homeopath must treat each patient according his or her unique symptom profile. By contrast, orthodox medicine's paint-by-number approach allows it to treat most cases of pneumonia as if they are the same.

Similar issues arise in relation to persons with multiple diagnoses. For example, it is still a convenient generalization to say that a person has asthma, constipation, and depression. To think of them as separate entities is an artificial construct of the medical mind. While regular medicine treats each of these three conditions as if they are independent and unrelated, the homeopath understands them to be different but interrelated facets of one larger constellation of problems, all of which are occurring to the same person. As such, successful homeopathic treatment requires that they be understood as the one problem that they are. It is a truly remarkable thing to witness the resolution of all facets of a person's health problems in response to a single well-chosen homeopathic medicine.

It is highly unlikely that any doctor has ever seen a patient who has had the same exact symptom pattern as another patient. No two illnesses are ever exactly alike. In this sense, the range of problems that homeopathy can treat is not limited because it does not rely on a diagnostic system that seeks to group patients into artificial categories. Each patient is taken at face value. All symptoms, warts, quirks, and characteristics are assumed to be part of the greater whole, and all symptoms, by definition, occur within the context of the individual and his or her life circumstances.

Homeopaths have the unique advantage of being able to treat the patient before a conventional diagnostic conclusion has been reached. Regular doctors, on the other hand, can waste valuable time trying to determine "what the patient has" before treatment can begin. Having been programmed by mainstream medical culture to think in like manner, patients often ask me "What do you think it is, doc? What do I have?" Without trying to be glib, I usually reply that, "You have what you just told me you have."

My intent is to convey to them that their own detailed descriptions of their problems is far more revealing than any diagnostic label. And those descriptions will be of greatest value in helping me choose a homeopathic medicine. This can be a hard concept for many patients to grasp. It is natural to want to know what illness one has—as if that label will magically lead to a solution. Unfortunately, this is often not the case.

The range of problems treatable with homeopathy is almost limitless. It is effective for acute illnesses like colds, fevers, viral conditions, coughs, flu, bronchitis, pneumonia, bladder infections, prostate infections, gallbladder attacks, hepatitis, and so on. Since mainstream medicine has so little to offer, homeopathy is especially valuable in terms of its ability to address chronic disease. I have seen it help migraines, arthritis of all types, insomnia, asthma, allergies, back pain, skin conditions, constipation, indigestion, infertility, and more. Homeopathy is also an excellent form of treatment for injuries like cuts, bruises, sprains, strains, burns, insect stings, and even head injuries and concussions. Last but not least, homeopathy is the medicine *par excellence* for mental and emotional problems like anxiety, depression, anger and rage issues, self-esteem issues, grief, jealousy, poor concentration, lack of mental focus, learning disabilities, phobias, and much more.

This is not to say that other methods are not needed or not helpful. The setting of a fractured bone is best handled by an orthopedic doctor. But homeopathy can be invaluable when it comes to treating the pain, inflammation, and swelling that accompanies that break. It can also be used to ensure that the break heals in a timely manner.

It is also true that there are limits to homeopathic treatment. As a general rule, the more long standing and chronic an illness is, the harder it is to treat. Similarly, the deeper an illness is, the more of a challenge it poses to the prescriber. Illnesses like Parkinson's disease, insulin dependent diabetes, schizophrenia, and cancer can benefit from homeopathic treatment but are unlikely to be cured once and for all.

Whether used in a primary or adjunct role, homeopathy can be of benefit in almost all situations. How it is used depends upon the circumstance. For example, although it is not impossible, homeopathy is unlikely to be able to reverse a cancer. But it can be quite helpful in reducing symptoms, improving vitality, and minimizing side effects for patients undergoing conventional cancer treatment. The quality of life of many cancer patients treated by orthodox means can suffer tremendously. As was the case when my mother became debilitated by cancer therapy, homeopathy made a world of a difference.

CHAPTER 3

Some Homeopathic Case Histories

> *What homeopathy has shown to be true a century ago is true today, for symptoms of disease and symptoms of drugs (remedies) do not change and that is the rock on which the basis of homeopathy rests.*
> –Garth Boericke, MD (1929)

The majority of physical health problems, both acute and chronic, can benefit from homeopathic care. By acute, I mean those ailments that spring up seemingly out of nowhere and are not part of the everyday experience of the patient. The common cold, flu, bronchitis, conjunctivitis, ear infections, bladder infections, and viral exanthems like chicken pox and measles, are examples of acute conditions. Once resolved, it is expected that acute conditions will not result in ongoing symptoms that continue to plague the patient.

Chronic ailments are, by definition, expected to continue, whether in continuous or episodic form. Arthritis, asthma, allergies, warts, sciatica, dysmenorrhea, ovarian cysts, bedwetting, and multiple sclerosis are examples of chronic conditions. Although migraines are seemingly discrete events, they are considered chronic due to the fact that they occur within the context of a series of similar events, which, when taken as a whole, constitute the chronic illness called migraine headaches. Asthma and allergies can be of a similar episodic nature and, in such cases, can be considered acute flare-ups of chronic ailments.

One way to understand the relationship between acute and chronic conditions is to note the fact that conventional treatment of an acute episode of asthma or migraines is not likely to prevent the condition from returning. In fact, as homeopaths will tell you, suppressive symptomatic treatment of acute episodes is likely to reinforce the chronicity of a problem and may even lead to entirely new health problems.

Homeopathic treatment for acute illness

I would like to share an assortment of brief case histories from my medical practice in order to give the reader a sense of the scope of homeopathic healing. I'll begin with examples of some acute ailments. Acute illnesses can be mild to severe and can last from days to weeks depending on the nature of the problem.

A case of a violent cough

A high school student already under my care consulted me one day for a nasty cough. What first began looking like a "stomach bug" with "vomiting and dry heaves" morphed over the course of several days into a "nasty cough." The cough, which had gone on for two weeks, was very dry and occurred in long, drawn out aggressive fits. The cough would make him gag and he had to hold his abdomen while coughing. I was interested to find out that the intensity of the cough had triggered a nosebleed on several different occasions. A short course of prednisone prescribed by his regular doctor had little impact on the cough. The prolonged awful experience had left him exhausted.

To conventional medicine, this is a difficult case with few options to offer other than supportive measures. The patient had already taken prednisone, a drug of last resort that doctors prescribe when they don't know what else to do. To a homeopath, this is a relatively straightforward case involving a well-known symptom pattern. Based upon the vomiting, the violent paroxysms of coughing that led to nosebleeds, and the patient's need to hold his abdomen while coughing, I prescribed a few doses of a homeopathic medicine. (Remedy choice?[10])

The young man's mother called a week later to report that, "He did very well. He was almost without cough by the next day." Although the cough was seemingly gone, it had made a slight comeback just that morning. I instructed her to give him two more doses of the remedy. The cough never returned.

A case of a young boy with croup

I received a call from the mother of a five year-old boy under my care. He had been up the past two nights with a croupy sounding cough. The mother, who has some knowledge of homeopathy, had already tried the classic trio of remedies indicated for croup. In the following order of succession, she had given him *Aconitum, Spongia,* and *Hepar sulph*—to no avail.

"He hasn't been hungry for the past three days." The cough is persistent and gets worse whenever he tries to lie down. His voice is a "little hoarse." He has a temperature of 100 degrees but sits on the couch under blankets, acting as if he feels chilly. Nevertheless, cold things seem to soothe his symptoms, "He wants freeze pops." Of great interest to me was the fact that he had repeatedly vomited up large amounts of mucus during his coughing spells.

The details of this case alerted me to a homeopathic medicine that is known to fit coughs that resemble croup, that are quieted by consuming cold things, and are associated with the production of a tremendous amount of mucus. The mother drove over to my office to pick up a few doses of a homeopathic medicine that I had selected. (Remedy choice?[11])

I received a phone call the next day. "I gave him the remedy when we got in the car and within ten minutes he stopped coughing. He's fine; it was a miracle! He's out riding his bike. Before this, he was on the couch for days."

Note how two different homeopathic medicines were used for the two different cough cases. This is the defining feature of homeopathic care. Each and every prescription is tailored to the individual specifics of the case. Although there may be similarities, no two cases are exactly alike. It is critical, therefore, that both patient and practitioner be observant and attuned to the details of all symptoms, which serve as clues in determining the correct remedy. Compare this to the one-size-fits-all approach of conventional medicine. The same need for individualization applies to the following two cases of mononucleosis, each of which required a different homeopathic medicine.

A case of mono with a sore throat

James was a college student who had been sick for a week. He tested positive for mononucleosis the day before consulting me. Most of his symptomatology focused on his throat. Swallowing was painful, he complained of a "bad taste," and there were white deposits on his tonsils. When I asked about the taste, he described it as "metallic."

The glands below his jawline were swollen. Breathing deeply caused him to cough. His nose was stuffed up and his ears felt plugged. He had a fever the day before. When I asked if he felt warm or chilly, he answered, "I wake sweating all over, warm and cold." Looking to confirm a suspicion I had for a potential remedy for James, I asked if he had been salivating much. "I'm spitting a lot. My pillow can get wet when I sleep."

James was manifesting the symptom picture of a common homeopathic medicine used for, among other things, sore throats and mononucleosis. The typical profile includes a bad taste in the mouth, a tendency to salivate heavily, and temperature instability that causes the person to feel warm, then cold, and then warm again. I instructed him to take three doses of the remedy per day for two days. (Remedy choice?[12])

On day six I received a call from James' mother who reported that he had recovered rapidly. He had no more sore throat, fever, sweats, swollen glands, bad taste, or salivating. "Most of his symptoms are gone! He's only a little tired. Thank you!"

To be clear, there is no effective conventional medical treatment for mononucleosis. The condition can sometimes take weeks, even months, to fully resolve on its own. Fortunately, homeopathy can be a godsend in such cases. I have seen homeopathy promote rapid recovery from mononucleosis on many occasions. Homeopathy can also work wonders for those who have never felt quite the same since contracting mononucleosis.

A case of mono with enormously swollen tonsils
Like the preceding case, the symptoms of mono in this case centered on the throat, but in a completely different way. When I first met Hamid, his father sat across from me in the consulting room acting as translator. As he explained, it wasn't due to a language barrier, "He can't speak because of his swollen tonsils."

A week earlier at college, Hamid had noticed swollen glands on the sides of his neck. His neck felt sore and he felt tired. The next day he developed a 101.5 degree fever and the tonsil on the left side of his throat began to swell. The left ear hurt on swallowing and his left temporomandibular joint (TMJ) was sore when he tried to open his mouth. I made note of the peculiar fact that it was painful to swallow liquids but he was able to tolerate cold oatmeal made with cold milk.

Hamid tested positive for mono and, in spite of the fact that he had been taking an antibiotic and a steroid (dexamethasone), his left tonsil grew larger with each successive day. To make matters worse, Hamid's right tonsil started to swell the day before our consultation. At this point, he was barely able to whisper. His left tonsil was about the size of a golf ball and it appeared to be almost completely obstructing his throat.

Naturally, I was very concerned. Hamid's swollen tonsils were not responding to state-of-the-art medical care. I wanted to help but had to proceed with great caution. His symptom pattern reflected the profile of a well-known remedy, which is given to people who develop left-sided symptoms that then spread to the right. The same remedy is known for sore throats that are aggravated by swallowing liquids and feel better from swallowing solid foods and cold things. I prescribed low doses (6C) of this homeopathic medicine to be taken three times per day for two days. (Remedy choice?[13])

Five days later, I received a call from Hamid himself. He was able to speak and I was hearing his voice for the very first time. "I'm a lot better. The swelling is almost gone. I'm going back to school today." Here we see another example of the power of homeopathy and its ability to handle a serious condition that conventional medicine was unable to help. Who knows what might have happened if Hamid had not received proper care. He may have wound up in the emergency room, perhaps needing a tracheotomy in order to breathe. Thankfully, that was not necessary.

Homeopathic treatment for chronic illness

The true strength of homeopathy lies in its ability to successfully treat chronic illness. This is quite the remarkable claim given the fact that conventional medicine is unable to cure a single chronic disease. At best it manages to control the symptoms of chronic illness, which is why medications for asthma, allergies, arthritis, and high blood pressure, for example, must be taken indefinitely. When those medicines are discontinued, the suppressive effect is removed, thus allowing symptoms to return.

Homeopathy, on the other hand, can often reverse chronic disease without suppressing symptoms and without requiring the patient to take medicines for the rest of his or her life. Let's take a look at a few more case histories involving a variety of chronic illnesses.

A severe case of atopic dermatitis

Starting with the most superficial of physical health problems, but not necessarily the simplest, homeopathy can be effective in treating all sorts of skin problems. I have seen it help patients with eczema, psoriasis, dermatitis, poison ivy, herpes, shingles, styes, ulcers, boils, hives, and much more.

Susan is a 52 year-old woman who consulted me about an intensely itchy skin rash that covered both arms, her neck, and parts of her face. She had eczema as a child, experienced a brief respite from skin troubles from ages twelve through eighteen, followed by mild recurrences of rashes on her hands that would always respond positively to corticosteroid skin cream applications. She also had swelling around the eyes that had been diagnosed as peri-orbital edema. Unfortunately, over the past two years her overall condition had spiraled out of control.

At her wits' end, she was willing to try anything doctors had to offer. By the time she reached me she was taking Benadryl for the itch, ibuprofen as an anti-inflammatory measure, a sedative called Lorazepam to treat the underlying stress that might be contributing to the rash, an immunosuppressive drug called Tacrolimus (normally used to prevent rejection of transplanted organs), a topical antibiotic cream called Mupirocin, and a topical steroid called Desoximetasone—all to little avail. The rash continued to rage on.

Clues of interest to me as a homeopathic doctor included the fact that Susan's rash was dry, red, irritated, and extremely itchy. The itch was worse under the covers in bed at night, causing her to scratch until she bled. When I asked about her temperature preferences, she explained that she tended to be very cold. She wore "a fleece and warm clothes inside the house all the time." The itch was disrupting her sleep and she was becoming increasingly "discouraged" about the prospect of getting any relief.

After prescribing a couple different homeopathic remedies to little effect, I settled on a third prescription, which began to turn the case around almost overnight. This medicine is known to fit people who have a generally pessimistic outlook on life and skin conditions that involve intense itchiness. Persons who need this remedy often report feeling very chilly and sensitive to cold temperatures. (Remedy choice?[14])

Two weeks after taking the medicine she reported, "The rash is almost gone. I'm very pleased. I'm just a little itchy." At five weeks, both the rash and itch were completely gone and the swelling around her eyes was lessening. "I'm so much improved, it's crazy!" Four months later, after repeating the remedy at intervals on three separate occasions, all of Susan's symptoms were gone. She had discontinued the use of all of her medications. She even reported that her chilliness had become less noticeable. She continues to be well to this day.

A woman with an assortment of female health problems

Homeopathy also has a well-established track record for treating women's health issues. Over the years, I have used it to successfully treat menstrual disorders like pre-menstrual symptoms, pain and cramping, heavy bleeding, irregular cycles, and amenorrhea (premature cessation of cycles). I have seen it help ovarian cysts, bladder infections, infertility, tendency to miscarriage, hormonally related mood disorders, the whole range of pregnancy-related issues, and menopausal symptoms including hot flashes and diminishing libido. One very common and relatively unrecognized female health problem is the long-term physical and emotional effects of prolonged birth control use. Homeopathy can work miracles by restoring normal hormonal balance in those who suffer from such effects. The following case involved several interrelated female health problems.

Tina is a thirty year-old woman who presented to me with recurrent vaginal yeast infections that started when she was in college. In addition, she had several genital herpes outbreaks in recent years, and a tendency to develop cold sores on her lips over the prior ten years. She also had a chronic vaginal discharge that would burn the skin. Most distressing of all were her frequent episodes of anal fissures, which were painful and could bleed.

She had tried everything from antifungal drugs to topical steroids to anti-yeast diets. Tina explained that all the symptoms combined were a significant impediment to her love life and tended to make sex a painful experience. In addition, she complained of being generally irritable, especially toward her husband and children.

I prescribed a well-known homeopathic remedy called *Sepia* because it matched a lot of her complaints. It seemed to work for a time but, eventually, the symptoms began to return. In the meantime, she had taken an antibiotic for a tooth infection that had become very irritated and painful. I chose another medicine also known to cover many of the symptoms that she described. This medicine is known to help skin symptoms that are very irritating and is also indicated for pain caused by sex. In addition, it is known for its great mental irritability. (Remedy choice?[15])

Soon after taking the remedy, Tina developed a head cold and a rash across her lower abdomen. Within a week, the rash faded and all her chronic symptoms had cleared up too. "Sex has been painless and I'm not angry." Three months after first taking the medicine she reported continued progress with almost no skin symptoms. "I'm happy. I'm really good."

A case of degenerative arthritis and migraine headaches

Julia is a forty-seven year old married woman with multiple chronic debilitating health problems. She has a long-standing history of migraines dating back to her early twenties. The migraines usually begin on waking from sleep. "It feels like my brain is too big for my skull." There is usually a "sticking pain" in one eye and the headaches make her "completely nauseous." Once she has a migraine, she becomes very sensitive to light and the smell of perfumes. Nowadays, they tend to occur anywhere from once every two weeks, to as frequently as twice per week.

In addition to the migraines, doctors have given Julia a diagnosis of degenerative arthritis of the cervical spine (mainly in the neck area). She describes neck pain "like a pole jammed up into the back of my skull. Now it's gone into my shoulders. I carry my stress in my neck." There is a history of a car accident involving whiplash, but Julia is uncertain as to whether that was when her troubles began. She takes several different drugs on an as-needed basis for neck and migraine pain.

Julia also has a number of lesser complaints, including night sweats, arthritic pain in her left foot, and rosacea. All of her symptoms combine to limit her daily activities in significant ways.

The specific details of headache pain can oftentimes provide useful clues that point to a homeopathic prescription—and sometimes not. In Julia's case, I took note of the fact that her favorite foods included strong spicy flavored foods, chocolate chip cookies, and chocolate milkshakes. She acknowledged having a stronger than average thirst. When I asked about fears, she noted that she was afraid of cancer and thunderstorms. When I asked about her temperament, Julia said, "I'm super perceptive. I have premonitions. I know things before I'm told of them. I'm very sympathetic." Based largely upon this information, I prescribed two doses of a homeopathic remedy. (Remedy choice?[16])

Three weeks later, at her follow-up visit, Julia reported having a "massive headache" for the first two days after taking the remedy. That was followed by a "good sense of well-being. I feel like myself again. As crazy as it sounds, my neck doesn't bother me. My husband is amazed!" She was doing so well that I decided not to give her another dose of the medicine. She willingly agreed.

One month later, she noted that she still felt good. "I snow-shoed eight miles and only had a twinge in my neck!" Her left foot was less painful and her rosacea was a little better, too. She had discontinued all of her conventional medications. Although her night sweats had been improved, she felt like she was "slipping a little" because they had acted up again over the past week. We decided together that it was time to take a couple more doses of the same remedy.

A month later, Julia reported, "I have no headaches or neck aches in spite of life's stressors. I'm fine. My friends are amazed. It's nothing short of a miracle!" She has continued to do well in the two years since I first saw her.

While allopathic diagnoses can feel to some like a lifelong prison sentence, it doesn't always have to be that way. The label, "degenerative arthritis," sounds rather grim and tends to give people the impression that they must learn to live with the pain. Largely because of our cultural indoctrination into materialistic thinking, we tend to believe doctors' explanations when we see concrete evidence, like an x-ray showing decay of the cervical vertebrae. But as this case illustrates, the reason given by conventional doctors for pain does not always turn out to be true. After all, there are lots of folks in the world who have no symptoms at all in spite of the fact that their x-rays would reveal similar arthritic abnormalities.

A case of exophthalmic hyperthyroidism
The power of homeopathy to change the course of one's life becomes abundantly clear when patients who were destined for the knife become well enough to no longer need surgery. I have seen homeopathy resolve gall bladder attacks, carpal tunnel syndrome, ovarian cysts, recurrent tonsillitis, chronic back pain, chronic ear infections and, in the case below, hyperthyroidism. Many were spared the trauma of surgical intervention.

Deborah is a fifty-one year old woman who consulted me for her recent diagnosis of an overactive thyroid. Previous health problems including insomnia and asthma seemed to escalate with the onset of her hyperthyroidism. New symptoms included heart racing and anxiousness.

Looking for potential factors that might have led to the development of her hyperthyroid condition, she noted that she had been taking daily HCG injections during the month preceding the onset of the problem. HCG (human chorionic gonadotropin) is a hormone produced during pregnancy that speeds metabolism and breaks down fat. Deborah had lost fifteen pounds while trying out this latest weight loss method, one of many such potentially dangerous weight loss fads offered by both conventional and alternative doctors.

She had been prescribed a beta-blocker for her palpitations, but the first dose triggered a severe asthma attack. Deborah was also given a prescription for the drug, methimazole, often used as the first line of defense in treating hyperthyroidism in the hope of avoiding having to surgically remove the thyroid gland. After her experience with the beta blocker, Deborah chose not to take the methimazole and decided to consult me instead.

What was interesting to me as a homeopathic prescriber was the fact that she also complained of hoarseness of her voice. "I'm dry as hell." On examination, there appeared to be a lump in her thyroid region, but her regular doctor had told her "it was only just fat." I noticed that her eyes were slightly bulging out. She acknowledged that she had been aware of this over the past couple years. Exophthalmia, or protruding eyeballs, is a symptom often associated with thyroid disorders.

The combination of symptoms including dryness of the throat, hoarse voice, asthma, overactive thyroid, and protruding eyeballs alerted me to a possible solution. Armed with this information, I chose a homeopathic medicine known to fit this unusual pattern of symptoms. I told her to take two doses and strongly advised that she discontinue the HCG shots. (Remedy choice?[17])

When she returned three weeks later, Deborah reported the following. "Within a few days, I felt my left eye recede inward, then the right eye later that same day. My husband and mother confirmed this. I feel more normal. I can close my eyes tight again." More importantly, all the hyperthyroid symptoms had virtually disappeared. There were no asthma symptoms and no heart racing. "The dryness is gone. I'm less anxious. I'm sleeping ten hours per night, that's unprecedented!" I took this as a positive sign of recuperation given her prior overactive thyroid-induced insomnia. In the following months, we repeated the prescription one more time (two more doses), and all has gone well since.

Some critics claim that homeopathic medicines only work as placebos, which, to their way of thinking, explains why homeopathy has a reputation for helping people with emotional problems. Here we have a case involving clear-cut organic pathology that would likely have necessitated surgical intervention. It is worth noting that the exophthalmia was unlikely to have ever resolved, even under the best of conventional treatment.

A case of multiple sclerosis

I first met Maryanne over fifteen years ago when she was struggling with extreme fatigue during her second pregnancy. Her first pregnancy had been quite traumatic. After being given an epidural injection for pain during labor she felt the whole right side of her body begin to "jerk." A few weeks after delivering her child, she began to experience trouble walking. "My legs weren't coordinated." To make a long story short, what was initially diagnosed as low back pain and treated with physical therapy eventually morphed into a full-blown diagnosis of multiple sclerosis (MS).

Maryanne's lower extremities became numb and tingly. As it progressed up her legs, her feet completely lost all feeling. She also developed severe headaches and debilitating fatigue. One night she awoke to find that she could not move her arms or hands. These symptoms and many others had waxed and waned over the ensuing three years since her first pregnancy. Each flare-up of MS symptoms would begin with pain on the right side of her body, in the same distribution as the original muscle jerking that she experienced after the epidural.

She was now consulting me because, although the first couple months of her current pregnancy had gone well, she was now experiencing a flare of her right-sided symptoms along with a noticeable increase in fatigue. She was understandably worried about what the future of this pregnancy, labor, and delivery might bring.

The simplest explanation for Maryanne's troubles was that the epidural had triggered her MS. Of course, orthodox medicine recognizes no such etiology for MS. Fortunately, there is a homeopathic medicine that is indicated for both puncture wounds and problems that result from injuries to the nerves. I reasoned that an epidural, which involves the insertion of a needle into a nerve-rich part of the body, satisfies both conditions of the remedy. I prescribed two doses in 30C potency. (Remedy choice?[18])

One month later, Maryanne reported that the next morning after taking the remedy she had a full-blown attack of MS numbness. It was unusual in that it came on very quickly, there was no pain, and there was less incoordination than normal. As the numbness gradually diminished over the following two weeks, her fatigue lifted. "I'm not having extreme exhaustion. I feel very level. I don't feel blah or depressed anymore. I've had no insomnia at all." We decided that she should not repeat the medicine at that time because she was already progressing in a positive direction.

Five weeks later Maryanne said, "I had all the signs of a flare-up coming but nothing happened. This is extremely unusual. I've had oodles of energy. I've had nothing since, no numbness, no pain. I feel fantastic." We opted again to do nothing. One month later, Maryanne's water broke and labor proceeded without complication. "My delivery was fabulous."

In the fifteen years since, Maryanne has had a few brief, mild flare-ups of MS—nothing nearly as bad as when we first began working together. With the help of two additional homeopathic medicines, *Natrum muriaticum* and *Causticum*, she eventually achieved full resolution of all MS symptoms. She now leads a normal life and has not experienced any MS-related issues in over five years.

In a case like this, it took sustained commitment over time in order to achieve maximum benefit. I have seen similar results with other neurologic diseases, including some conditions that have stumped neurologists. Neurologic disorders are complex and varied, oftentimes defying conventional disease classification. For homeopathy, however, it is not necessary to arrive at a clear diagnosis in order to achieve therapeutic success. I have successfully used homeopathy to treat Bell's palsy, trigeminal neuralgia, sciatica, and chronic Lyme disease.

Some neurologic diseases run very deep and success in such cases is a relative term. For some conditions, like Parkinson's disease, it would be considered a success to diminish the intensity of symptoms, or to slow down or arrest the progression of pathology. Conventional Parkinson's medications notoriously lose their effectiveness over time as the illness advances, thus necessitating changes in drug doses and drug combinations as a way of keeping up with the disease. I have a patient with Parkinson's who experiences psychiatric symptoms with each change of his drug regimen. Homeopathic interventions have stabilized him every time, have kept the side effects to a minimum, and have kept his Parkinson's stable, prolonging the duration of effectiveness of his conventional drugs.

Homeopathy for mental and emotional health

Another true strength of homeopathy lies in its ability to treat mental, emotional, and psychiatric illness. Few people understand the power of homeopathy in this realm—until they actually see it or experience it for themselves. When we come to realize that mind and body are one, and that most physical illness has its origins in emotional disturbances, then we can also see how homeopathic treatment of psychological issues can treat and prevent physical illness at its roots.

For example, I have had great success helping kids with nightmares and/or night terrors. Such children can dramatically disrupt family life. Their fears may require elaborate bedtime rituals in order to get them to sleep. Even older children may need to sleep in their parents' rooms on a nightly basis in order to cope with their fears. A well-chosen homeopathic prescription can eliminate the nightmares and allow the child to overcome his or her fears, thus restoring peace to the household.

Anxieties, phobias, and psychological complexes are stubborn problems that some can spend a lifetime trying to overcome. Years in therapy may be needed just to enable a person to cope with issues that, although largely invisible to most, are very real and can wreak havoc in their lives. I have seen a good homeopathic prescription virtually eliminate such issues in a matter of weeks or months. It may sound too good to be true, but any homeopathic practitioner can testify to this fact.

The amazing thing is that even very specific fears like fear of heights, flying, thunderstorms, spiders, or snakes can be addressed with a correct homeopathic prescription. More generally speaking, homeopathy can be invaluable in treating anxiety disorders, panic attacks, depression, suicidal thoughts, attention deficit issues, post-traumatic stress disorder, manic depression, and much more. Even issues that we believe to be ideal for psychotherapeutic intervention will respond well to a good homeopathic prescription. I have seen it benefit patients with motivational problems, low self-esteem issues, social anxieties, grief-related problems, and trust and anger issues.

Homeopathy can be of most help when the core psychological issues of the patient are identified and confirmed. Psychological complexes such as "I've always been a failure," "Nobody loves me," "I always have to be the best at what I do," and "I feel like people are judging me," once identified, can provide the key to solving homeopathic cases. Successful treatment can release the patient from the lifelong grip of such a complex. This first case illustrates one such psychologically debilitating complex.

A case of a young man who feels like he doesn't belong
I first met Andrew when he was a senior in high school. He was seeking my help for depression. He estimated that he had been "really down" for at least a couple of years. A yearlong course of an antidepressant had "only worked for a month."

Here, in his own words, is how Andrew described his struggles. "No matter what I do, my mind tells me I'm a failure. I feel like I'll never fit in or belong. It's demotivating. I try to act normally. I don't want to seem like a freak." When I asked, Andrew admitted to having occasional suicidal thoughts. "They come and go at real low points. I wouldn't have to worry about being such a failure anymore."

Of great interest to me as a homeopath was the fact that Andrew had been receiving allergy shots on a weekly basis for the prior three years. The purpose was to treat his seasonal allergies, which manifested mainly as sinus congestion. In fact, he had developed an anaphylactic reaction to his allergy injection just two weeks before his first visit with me. The resulting wheezing was treated with prednisone.

My mind immediately went to a familiar homeopathic remedy that seemed to match Andrew's complaints quite well. It is a medicine for those who suffer from lack of self-esteem, and who specifically complain of the feeling of not fitting into their social surroundings. Homeopathic reference books reveal that this medicine is also known for its sinus congestion and tendency to develop asthma.

Amazingly, it is also a remedy used for the adverse effects of vaccinations. Allergy shots are, in essence, a form of vaccination repeated over and over again. In fact, this remedy is known for its ability to treat cases of vaccine-induced asthma. I was concerned about Andrew's recent allergic reaction and the possibility that the shots might be leading him down the road to chronic asthma. I explained this to him and suggested that it might be in his best interest to discontinue the allergy shots. I prescribed two doses of this homeopathic medicine after he assured me that he was safe and that I did not have to be worried about his potential for self-harm. (Remedy choice?[19])

Andrew returned two weeks later with the following news. "I'm definitely not being so self-doubting anymore about how I look. I haven't had any down moods. My girlfriend says I'm more outgoing, less cautious." He had taken my advice and had discontinued the allergy shots. "I'm starting to feel a little stuffed up." I asked and he denied having any suicidal thoughts. I sent him home with two more doses of the remedy to be taken when he felt the need.

One month later, he told me that he had taken the remedy after two weeks because he felt down again. "I feel like it's working. I'm not depressed; no thoughts of wishing I wasn't here. I feel like I'm growing out of things (meaning, his psychological issues). Failure doesn't worry me as much" However, he still felt that he wasn't sufficiently motivated about his schoolwork. I prescribed two more doses.

Over the next few months we repeated the same medicine several times, once in a stronger potency. Six months after starting treatment Andrew was like a new person. His depression was gone and his motivation had been restored. He had developed "new study habits" and was "more organized" about his work. He was not experiencing nasal congestion in spite of having ended his allergy shots. Andrew went on to attend college and now runs a new business of his own.

The important lesson here is that medical interventions aimed at treating physical problems can also impact the psyche. In this case, I believe that the allergy shots were the primary contributing factor to Andrew's depression. While conventional medicine looks the other way when it comes to such phenomena, homeopaths are trained to identify the connections. When we consider that modern children receive far more vaccinations now than did earlier generations, the implications regarding their long-term mental and emotional health are staggering.

A case of a young girl who expresses her stress through her skin

The following case illustrates the undeniably powerful connection between psychological difficulties and physical health problems. A mother brought her seven year-old daughter to me seeking help for a condition called molluscum contagiosum. Conventional medicine attributes this wart-like skin eruption to a virus, but has little to offer in terms of treatment. In fact, the dermatologist had told Becky to "leave it alone," reassuring her that it would eventually go away.

Initially, there was a cluster of molluscum on Becky's left arm. Later, more clusters appeared on her left knee and shin. During this same time frame she had also developed psoriasis behind her ears. It was now a year and a half since she first contracted the molluscum. Becky's mother explained to me that, "She seems to express herself through her skin. When she's happy, her skin glows. When she's troubled, she gets skin symptoms. She does a lot of internal processing"

When I asked Becky what she thought about the molluscum she said, "They're disgusting." I asked mom to tell me more about Becky. "She's deep. She thinks a lot. She doesn't like me to talk about her. Her father and I divorced three years ago. She handled it internally. She likes to be alone. She's a prolific reader."

After consulting my homeopathic reference books, I concluded that there were two solid remedy choices that might help Becky. *Thuja* is known for symptoms that appear on the left side of the body. It is also indicated for people who feel themselves to be "ugly." This is not an unusual feeling among those who have herpes or warts. But I chose the other possibility, which is a remedy that can help people who develop health problems as a result of internalizing their emotions. (Remedy choice?[20])

At the follow-up visit, Becky's mother reported that, "The molluscum was gone within three days. And that remedy was so good for her self-esteem. She has improved emotionally in a hundred ways." The psoriasis had cleared as well. Becky's own statement said it all, "I try to keep things in, but sometimes they come out."

As you can see, skin problems are not always just skin problems, and homeopathic treatment runs more than skin deep. The connection between Becky's skin and her psychological state is evident in this case. The skin is often a reflection of underlying health problems, including psychological issues. Homeopathy teaches us that most physical health problems have a deeper connection to the human psyche.

Conventional medicine does not acknowledge these types of mind-body relationships and, even if it did, it has neither the philosophical framework nor the practical means by which to manage them. This also explains why targeted treatment of localized symptoms often brings only temporary relief. It fails to get to the root of the problem, which is sometimes psychological and almost always systemic.

An explosive case of attention-deficit/hyperactivity disorder (ADHD)
When I first met James, he was almost completely oblivious of the fact that he was sitting in my consulting room. Instead, he was deeply absorbed in the action taking place on the screen of his portable video game. He alternatingly laughed, talked to himself, hit himself in the head, and shouted while violently shaking his game device. At one point he yelled, "kill, die!" as if the thing could hear him, and as if my presence meant nothing to him.

His mother explained that James, who was now in seventh grade, "gets very upset. He explodes when frustrated or if he is pushed to do something. He's a very smart kid but he doesn't want to do any work. He's a master of manipulating situations." When I finally managed to get James' attention, he acknowledged what his mother had described. "I flip out. I get really mad when people say stuff about me. I get in their face."

After teachers insisted that James needed medicine for his aggression, his mother sought psychiatric help. After taking three doses of the ADHD drug, Adderall, James "became depressed and talked about suicide." His mother was now looking to me for a safer alternative approach.

Our discussion brought additional facts to light. James needed to be in constant motion. "I hate a small room. If I don't have room for my body, I get agitated." In fact, he was very athletic. "All sports come easily to me." It turns out that James was musically talented, too. He enjoyed dancing and singing. Unfortunately, he also tended to engage in "high risk behaviors." He once fractured a clavicle while riding recklessly on his scooter. "I'm very daring."

Our conversation reminded me of a homeopathic medicine known for its intense restlessness and inability to sit still. Individuals who respond well to this medicine are also known to be very agile and musically inclined. Sports and music are great outlets for the tremendous pent up energy in these persons. I prescribed one moderately strong dose of this remedy to James. (Remedy choice?[21])

At the follow-up visit one month later, James' mother was very pleased. "Things are definitely better. I'm amazed. So many people notice a difference. The social worker notices drastic changes. He's stopping and thinking about things more—about himself and his future. He's more pleasant and less reactive. His anger is so much more manageable. He's actually doing his work at school. It's almost like a piece of his development had been missing." James agreed. "I know there's a change. I'm not getting angry as much."

Over the ensuing year, James was given four more doses of the same medicine. Although there were a few ups and downs, in that time he had seemingly grown up. "He's not hyper like he was. He's paying attention. He's planning ahead. His teachers see great progress." He was gradually "mainstreamed" into more suitable classes. He decided to take up guitar lessons. He was even becoming aware of personal hygiene. Repeat psychological testing revealed that he was no longer considered to be in the ADHD range. At one point, his mother noted, "He's ninety-nine percent better than he ever was."

This case illustrates how homeopathy can literally turn a person's life around. There is no telling what trouble James was headed for if he hadn't been able to get a handle on his wild energy. And we can't underestimate the positive difference this will make for James' future.

Contrary to what some think, the spectrum of attention deficit and hyperactivity disorders is not a fiction created by PhRMA. Granted, the label is overused and sometimes applied inappropriately to situations where kids act out in response to genuine external triggers. On the other hand, many kids with ADHD endure a great deal of very real suffering. Proper homeopathic intervention has the potential to reduce suffering and improve the quality of their lives.

Homeopathy for those who have "never been well since…"
Homeopathy is unique in that patients don't have to wait around for treatment until blood work and other tests confirm some suspected diagnosis. By contrast, more than a few conventional medical patients fail to meet the criteria for a specific diagnosis and, instead of receiving medical care, are referred from specialist to specialist in hope of discovering that elusive diagnostic label. Some of these patients are given a clean bill of health in spite of the fact that they still don't feel well. While all tests turn out to be normal, the patient, nevertheless, continues to suffer.

From a homeopathic perspective, there is a category of patients that are referred to as those who have "never been well since." These are the patients who can pinpoint an event in their lives that coincided with a downturn in their health. Such events vary greatly from person to person and represent physical or psychological turning points. Oftentimes the original event has long passed and, yet, the person will indicate that they have never been quite the same since that event. In spite of the fact that the original event may have been a medically diagnosable problem, subsequent examination or testing may no longer detect any problem.

For example, a patient may have contracted a case of bronchitis six months ago. Although the acute episode of bronchitis is long over, the person may complain of never having fully recovered. By conventional standards, there is no more bronchitis and, therefore, no problem left to treat. And yet, the person continues to feel poorly, perhaps complaining of fatigue or aches or even a lingering occasional cough.

The controversy over chronic Lyme disease is a case in point. The medical establishment insists that once a patient has been treated with antibiotics and lab values no longer indicate active Lyme disease, then there is nothing further to be done. This, in spite of the fact that many Lyme patients who have received the recommended drug treatment never return to their normal states of health. Some in the alternative medical community argue that these are the patients who have chronic Lyme disease. Mainstream medicine counters that this can't be so if lab tests indicate that a patient is no longer Lyme positive. Some holistic physicians have been called into question by mainstream medical authorities because they dare to claim that they can help patients with "chronic Lyme."

Around and around the debate over semantics goes. And that is precisely what it is—a dispute over the meaning of terminology, with both sides arguing over the existence of something called chronic Lyme disease. Meanwhile, the poor patients stuck in this diagnostic no man's land are ignored by the medical establishment and discouraged from seeking treatment from alternative healthcare practitioners.

Homeopaths, on the other hand, understand that the debate boils down to a question of semantics. They know that diagnostic labels are only stereotypes. While they don't ignore potentially helpful diagnostic information, they also don't place too much faith in the accuracy of diagnostic labels. To a homeopath, it doesn't matter if the diagnosis is unclear because it is the patient's story that counts most. If a patient reports having received the appropriate antibiotic treatment for Lyme disease and thereafter continues to struggle with a number of new health issues that weren't there before the Lyme diagnosis, then that is what a homeopath refers to as a patient who has "never been well" since Lyme. That is the bottom line, whether one labels such cases chronic Lyme disease or not.

There are many such patients that meet this description, who have recovered from the acute phase of an illness but have never returned to a normal state of health. Although the conventional medical model does not account for these patients and their circumstances, homeopathy has long recognized them as "never well since" cases. The good news is that there is homeopathic treatment available to them. This is made possible by the fact that homeopathy does not treat disease stereotypes. It approaches each person and his or her illness as a new and unique variation of the allopathic stereotype. Each case requires individualized care based upon the specific details of that case.

It comes as no surprise to a homeopath, then, when a person complains of having never been the same since contracting mononucleosis five years ago, or since breaking a bone from a fall off a bike. Some report never having been well since a death in the family, the loss of a job, or the breakup of a relationship. Many others can trace a decline in their health back to medical interventions, whether from drugs, surgeries, or diagnostic procedures. Literally anything can act as a trigger or a turning point—even good news. "I was so shocked when I won that million dollar lottery. I've been anxious and unable to sleep ever since."

A case of a young woman who has never been well since contracting the flu

Cheryl is a college student who had struggled with her health since coming down with the flu two years earlier. At the time, she developed fever, chills, aches, headache, fatigue, and a sore throat. After the fever and chills abated, she continued to feel tired and achy. She complained of malaise, "I don't want to do anything."

Several months later, she came down with strep throat. Antibiotic treatment cleared the strep but she continued to feel tired and achy. "My body always feels warm." Cheryl's mother thought that she was acting somewhat depressed ever since the original flu. Cheryl gradually improved, but not completely, until she caught a stomach bug six months later. This episode involved nausea, fever, chills, and vomiting. The unfortunate chain of adverse health events continued as she developed strep throat again. Yet another flu-like episode was diagnosed as Coxsackie virus. Not surprisingly, Cheryl's general health had declined over the course of those two years. She became increasingly fatigued and "unmotivated," and continued to complain of feeling unusually warm.

Further questioning revealed that Cheryl was a serious student. Her health had created an enormous mental and physical strain as she labored to keep up with her college coursework. She was also the kind of person who would go above and beyond the call of duty, often helping her sister, for example, with her problems. I asked if overextending herself like that was advisable given her condition. She replied, "I'd feel guilty otherwise."

A few additional clues helped confirm my suspicions regarding a potential remedy that might be of help to Cheryl. She admitted to being "sensitive to everything." She loved thunderstorms because they gave her a thrill. And she acknowledged that chocolate was her favorite treat. Based on this, along with the chronic fatigue triggered by the original flu, and the nature of her temperament, I prescribed a couple doses of a homeopathic medicine. (Remedy choice?[22])

One month later, Cheryl reported having had headaches during the first few days after taking the remedy. "Then everything else went away." The fatigue, body aches, and feverish feeling disappeared. "I'm not unmotivated. I have a lot more energy. School is good." Cheryl's father agreed, "She seems cheerier."

Over the course of the next six months, Cheryl experienced a couple of mild flare-ups of her symptoms. Each time, additional doses of the same remedy restored her back to general overall good health. She has had no acute illnesses in the two years since and, thanks to homeopathy, she is back to feeling like her old self again.

CHAPTER 4
Remedies and References

> *A homeopathic prescription is one which contains, in a subphysiological dose, the single remedy which produces all the symptoms, sensations, and a pathology or physiological disturbance similar to that of the disease for which the prescription is intended...*
>
> –George Royal, MD (1930)
>
> *What do we mean by the totality of symptoms? All the symptoms observed in a patient—both subjective and objective. It is the outwardly reflected image of the diseased state, and is the only condition to be recognized for removal and consequent restoration to health.*
>
> –Willis A Dewey, MD (1908)
>
> *A good way to study a symptom or a drug is to read, study, think; think, study, read...*
>
> –George Royal, MD (1930)

Homeopathic references

The vast storehouse of information accumulated by homeopathic practitioners over the past two hundred years is staggering. Without a photographic memory, no mere mortal is capable of retaining or recalling all of the data pertaining to thousands of homeopathic remedies and hundreds of thousands of symptoms. Thankfully, a great deal of that information has been carefully preserved in a wide variety of indispensable reference books.

I do not envy either the pioneers of homeopathy or my contemporary colleagues who have devoted endless hours of their time archiving, maintaining, and collating this monumental database of information. Homeopathic practitioners and patients the world over owe a tremendous debt of gratitude to these selfless individuals without whom homeopathy might be just a footnote in history. Julian Winston, whose *Heritage of Homœopathic Literature* is the definitive modern homeopathic bibliography, makes reference to the incompleteness of his work, which lists 915 volumes, by comparing it to an earlier bibliography.

> When T. L. Bradford compiled his *Homœopathic Bibliography* in 1892, he listed 872 authors and over 3,000 written works. His book covered only those works which had been printed in the USA until that time, although he did have a full listing of most of the foreign publications of Hahnemann's work. It is a valuable and unique volume, and long out of print. There is no such analogous volume for the works produced in the UK and for those authors whose works were not issued in an American printing.[23]

There are many "how to" books designed to guide laypersons in the use of homeopathic medicines in first aid situations. There are also many "principles and practice" books that are designed to instruct professionals in the art and science of homeopathic prescribing. But the reference books used by homeopathic practitioners—the ones that contain that vast storehouse of information—fall into two main categories. One type is called a *materia medica* and the other is known as a *repertory*.

Materia medicas contain information about each specific homeopathic remedy. Most are organized alphabetically according to the name of the remedy. Listed under the section for each homeopathic medicine one can learn about the many mental, emotional, and physical symptoms that it is associated with—the symptoms it is known to cause and to be able to treat. Much of the information contained in a *materia medica* comes from provings. Additional information comes from clinical observations made by practitioners who have documented the effective use of a medicine in treating specific symptoms. Information is also culled from toxicology reports of persons who have been accidentally poisoned. For example, symptoms that develop from a snake bite or spider bite can be found in a *materia medica* under the section for that specific snake or spider.

Dr. Hahnemann conducted the very first provings, and homeopaths and their students have continued his work ever since. A proving involves the administration of a homeopathically diluted substance to test subjects, also known as *provers*, who then carefully record all symptoms that emerge in response. Homeopathic provings are unique in that they are conducted on healthy test subjects who have very few baseline symptoms. Special care is taken to ensure that symptoms from the test substance are not confused with provers' baseline symptoms.

To maintain scientific integrity, provers are unaware of the homeopathic substance being tested. Some provings also include a placebo group. A remedy is administered on a daily basis until symptoms develop. Each prover documents his or her symptoms in great detail. This includes all physical, emotional, and mental symptoms that the prover experiences in both the short and longer term. The collective information gathered from the group of provers is then collated and analyzed. Some of the more reliable information, especially symptoms experienced by multiple provers, is eventually verified and accepted into the official *materia medica*.

Materia medicas vary in length, ranging from a single volume to many volumes. Perhaps the most famous *materia medica* is the one written by William Boericke, MD, originally published in 1901.[24] The 9th edition of his *Pocket Manual of Homœopathic Materia Medica* is still in widespread use today. Don't be fooled by the title; it contains over one thousand pages and references more than 1,300 homeopathic remedies. Larger *materia medicas* contain all available data on each given substance, while others contain only what the author believes to be the most pertinent information regarding a more limited choice of remedies. "Keynote" *materia medicas* are bare bones reference books that list the main features of a remedy and its uses. Keynote books are incomplete but can serve as useful learning tools and quick references.

Under the listing for a specific medicine in a *materia medica* one can find information about its source, its original proving, and the mental, emotional, and physical symptoms that it is known to be able to cause and, therefore, to treat. Symptoms are usually organized according to body part. One section contains all the eye symptoms, another contains the skin symptoms, and so on. There are often additional categories that contain vertigo symptoms, cough symptoms, fever, chill, and perspiration symptoms, and even sleep symptoms. The "Mind" section contains mental and emotional symptoms and characteristics. The "Generalities" or "Generals" section contains symptoms that apply to the person as a whole. Here you will find information about hunger, thirst, body temperature, weather sensitivities, and much more. One can differentiate a general symptom from a more specific symptom by the way a person verbalizes that symptom. For example, it is proper form to say, "I feel sleepy," or, "I can't tolerate hot humid weather," as opposed to, "my back hurts," or, "my cough is dry." If I am cold, it is considered a general. If my hands are cold, it is specific only to the hands.

Another important and relatively modern aspect of *materia medica* concerns the psychological profiles of remedies. James Tyler Kent, MD was a pioneer in the field. Kent's *Lectures on Homeopathic Materia Medica*,[25] published in 1905, took a decidedly more nuanced approach to describing remedy pictures, especially in terms of the characterological makeup of individuals who had responded best to certain remedies. His contribution was ahead of its time, well before the dawning of the contemporary psychological era.

It wasn't until the 1970's that Greek homeopath, George Vithoulkas, expanded upon Kent's efforts with his "essences" of homeopathic medicines.[26] The essences are descriptions of themes that run throughout remedy pictures, themes that are often expressed on both physical and psychological levels. In the symptom profile of *Nux vomica*, for example, one can discern a type of urgency that makes itself known on all levels. The type of person who could benefit from *Nux vomica* is one who is always in a hurry, anxious to complete the job as efficiently as possible. On the physical level, the same person may experience a strong painful urge to urinate, or the famous *Nux vomica* constipation, which is described as an "ineffectual urging" to stool. Urgency is the common theme.

Rajan Sankaran's *The Spirit of Homeopathy*[27] is a more recent contribution to the homeopathic literature. In it, Dr. Sankaran suggests that one can discern a "central disturbance" or "core delusion" in the symptom pictures of certain remedies. This delusion is a fixed or false belief that holds sway over the person, a central psychological complex from which most other emotional and physical pathology evolves. Sankaran's idea is that deep healing can be achieved by making sure that the homeopathic prescription is capable of addressing the core issue of the patient. For example, Sankaran describes the core issue of the remedy, *Lyssinum*, as a feeling...

> "... of having suffered wrong, being tormented, especially by one whom he has served, has been faithful to and is dependent on, thus creating an intense feeling of anger and rage..."[28]

From this central dilemma arise all other difficulties of the *Lyssinum* patient, both of a psychological and physical nature.

A number of similar contributions have been made to the *materia medica* by other contemporary homeopathic authors. Catherine Coulter, Frans Vermeulen, Jan Scholten, Jeremy Sherr, and Massimo Mangialavori are just a few such pioneers of the modern *materia medica*. The homeopathic *materia medica*, therefore, is always a work in progress. It evolves over the course of time, thanks to the contributions of practitioners and provers who have documented their experiences for the benefit of us all.

While the *materia medica* evolves with each new remedy contribution, homeopathy itself does not change. That is the fickle fate of conventional medicine, with its ever-shifting theories and protocols, brought to us by an increasingly unreliable body of corporate funded research. The *materia medica* evolves in the sense that it steadily accumulates new remedy information over the course of time. New data enriches the picture of old remedies, fills out the images of lesser-known remedies, and introduces valuable new remedies to the homeopathic pharmacy. The expanding nature of the *materia medica* does not alter the foundational principles of homeopathic practice, which have remained essentially the same since the time of Hahnemann. It does, however, increase the therapeutic options available to all homeopathic practitioners.

There is a distinct tendency for contemporary practitioners to rely too heavily on psychological profiling as a shortcut to prescribing. Because we live in a psychological age, it is understandable why this approach would be so appealing. While it is true that a patient's personality traits, emotional issues, fears, and character quirks can point directly to a correct homeopathic medicine, it is also true that these clues can lead one down the wrong path. This type of psychological profiling is highly subjective and open to individual interpretation. Additional clues of a non-psychological nature can be very important in confirming the choice of a remedy that one initially suspects based on characterological clues. It is important to strike a balance, one that utilizes all types of information and is not skewed in favor of any one dimension of a patient's case history.

It is important to understand that normal traits such as extroversion or introversion are not viewed as abnormal unless they are exaggerated to a point where they create difficulties for the person. Some individuals describe themselves as introverted and are perfectly happy being so. Others experience it as a burden that interferes with their pursuit of happiness. Such traits may still serve as clues to the homeopath, but are not expected to be altered by a correct remedy unless they constitute part of the problem in the first place.

The information contained in a *materia medica* can be overwhelming. Because they cannot be memorized, *materia medicas* are intended as reference books. However, one would not want to search through an entire *materia medica* in order to discover the remedies that are known to be associated with a fear of birds, for example. It is not practical to read through all the remedy listings to find the ones that have this specific fear. Fortunately, that is why we have *repertories*. While a *materia medica* is like a remedy dictionary, a repertory is essentially a symptom index.

One can look up thousands of symptoms in a repertory. Each symptom listed in a repertory is also called a *rubric*. Under each symptom listed, one can find the homeopathic medicines known to cause that symptom. For example, under the "mind" section of a repertory I can look up the rubric, "jealousy," where it will list the medicines known to fit the symptom of jealousy. As per the homeopathic principle of similars, those are the remedies that can be used to treat people who have issues with jealousy.

In 1900, James Tyler Kent, MD, released his *Repertory of Homœopathic Materia Medica*.[29] This monumental symptom index contained 1,349 pages and is still the standard against which all repertories are judged. It boggles the mind to think that Dr. Kent compiled this invaluable resource without the aid of modern technology and computing. Nowadays, the entire process is computerized, thus allowing the symptoms pertaining to new remedies and new provings to be easily added as they are discovered. Many have continued the tradition, both as conservators and innovators of the modern repertory. Dr. Jost Künzli von Fimmelsberg, David Warkentin, Dr. Jugal Kishore, and Roger van Zandvoort are just a few such luminaries who have dedicated their time to repertorial development.

If a patient tells me that he has a tickling cough that acts up at night, I can find out what remedies fit this symptom by looking in the repertory under the rubric, "Cough, tickling, night." As you can see, repertories are invaluable tools that help one sift through the enormous homeopathic database of symptoms. When I find that *Drosera* is one such remedy listed under that specific cough symptom, I can learn more about that remedy by reading about it in a *materia medica*. If I decide that it is a good fit, I may consider it for my patient.

Remember, symptoms are not the object of treatment in homeopathy. Symptoms serve only as clues. The cough symptom is a clue that leads me to consider the remedy, *Drosera*, which may or may not be a suitable medicine for the overall condition of my patient. *Reperto-*

ries help us find the various remedies that fit a particular symptom or symptoms, and *materia medicas* allow us to study the full picture of each individual remedy in order to choose the one that best fits the situation at hand.

Remedy pictures

Now I will briefly sketch a couple of remedy pictures to help the reader get a sense of what the information in a *materia medica* looks like. A typical remedy description begins with general information about the substance itself, what it is, and where it originates. A "mind" section that lists psychological traits of the remedy picture usually follows this. After this come subsections that list symptoms pertaining to different body parts and other categories such as generalities, vertigo, and so on.

Some *materia medicas* include a section on "modalities." Modalities are factors or influences that affect symptoms for better or for worse. In homeopathy, we say that a modality either "aggravates" or "ameliorates" a symptom. For example, one person may say that his asthma gets worse in hot humid weather, another says that her asthma is worse at 2am, and a third says that his acts up when he tries to lie down. In the first case, the modality is a weather factor, in the second, a time factor, and in the third, a positional factor.

Let's try a few more modality examples. One person's headaches tend to act up around 3pm, are aggravated by light, and ameliorated by lying in a warm bed. (Remedy choice?[30]) Another person's headaches are made worse by noise and motion, and soothed by cold compresses. (Remedy choice?[31]) You can see how these modalities can help paint a picture that distinguishes the first person's headaches from the second. It is not particularly helpful to a homeopath when a patient simply reports that he or she gets headaches. However, when a patient says that the headaches are worse before a rainstorm and feel better from walking around, that information can point directly to a remedy. (Remedy choice?[32])

Modalities serve as very important clues in homeopathy. They highlight the unique manner in which each person experiences his or her symptoms. They help differentiate one person's version of a symptom from another person's. This is yet another factor that differentiates homeopathy from regular medicine. Cookie-cutter diagnostic labels serve little purpose in homeopathy because they do not provide enough information to support an accurate prescription.

The following is a brief sketch of a commonly indicated homeopathic medicine.

Keynote Materia Medica: *Lycopodium clavatum*

SOURCE: This medicine is derived from the Club Moss, aka Wolf's Claw. It is prepared from the spores of the plant. In its natural form, the plant is relatively inert. Its medicinal properties become more apparent through provings in its potentized form.

MIND: The main theme that runs throughout this remedy is a need to overcompensate for a general feeling of lack of confidence. Internal feelings of inferiority are masked by displays of bravado. The person may act in an egotistical manner, for example, by bragging, while not admitting to his or her true feelings of inadequacy. Some patients display one aspect of these polar opposites more than the other, while others show signs of both. A common example is the child who acts shy at school but bossy at home where he frequently corrects his parents' statements and presumes to tell them when they are wrong.

Low self-esteem, cowardly
Avoidance of responsibility
Domineering, bullying
Fear of failure
Fear of new situations, fear of new people
Fear of public speaking, stage fright

GENERALS:

Right-sided symptoms (headache, ear infection, kidney stone, sore throat, etc.)

Symptoms begin on the right and then extend to the left or switch to the left

General aggravation from 4 to 8pm

General tendency to feel chilly but may also fit warm-blooded persons

Strong desire for sweets

GASTROINTESTINAL:

These patients tend to have a lot of digestive troubles

Gas, bloating, belching, and flatulence

Stomach feels full after eating small amounts

Large appetite, tendency to overeat

Liver/gallbladder disorders, hepatitis, cholecystitis

MODALITIES:

Worse right side

Worse 4 to 8pm

Worse pressure of clothing on abdomen, worse belt around waist

Worse from embarrassment

Better from belching

Sore throat ameliorated by warm drinks

RELATIONSHIPS:

Complementary to *Lachesis, Chelidonium*

Often indicted in sequence with *Calcarea carbonica, Sulphur*

Compare to *Anacardium, Argentum nitricum, China*

    This is a very brief summary of details culled from the much more extensive list of symptoms attributed to *Lycopodium* in the *materia medica*. Note that the person who needs this remedy can exhibit both cowardliness and cockiness. Think of the cowardly lion in *The Wizard of Oz* and even the Wizard himself. Also note that some symptoms are repeated under Modalities and Generals. While the *Lycopodium* headache may specifically be worse from 4 to 8pm, the person who needs *Lycopodium* may also feel generally worse as a whole during the same time frame. Also note that while some who need this remedy tend to overeat, and while others feel full from the slightest amount, certain individuals may exhibit both tendencies.

The following is a brief summary of another commonly prescribed homeopathic remedy.

Keynote Materia Medica: *Sepia officinalis*

SOURCE: AKA *Sepia succuss*. This medicine is derived from the ink of the cuttlefish, which is a mollusk related to the squid and octopus. The animal can discharge ink from its ink sac when it feels threatened, creating a type of smokescreen enabling its escape. The ink is the same dark brown pigment known to many as India ink.

MIND: The main idea behind this remedy is a hormonal imbalance that tends to manifest as a state of physical and/or emotional stasis. It is prescribed mainly, although not exclusively, for women who display such tendencies. People who need *Sepia* tend to complain of a type of worn out depression characterized by apathy, indifference, and a lack of interest in activities traditionally associated with nurturing children and raising a family. This may present as an impatient irritability toward husband and children, an aversion to sexual contact, or a need to get away from the home. A good example of this type of hormonally induced state is post-partum depression.

Apathy, a "blah" state of neutrality
Indifferent and/or irritable toward family
Aversion to "domesticity"
Aversion to husband, children, and home
Prefers to be away from the home, would rather be working
    or exercising
Involuntary weeping for no clear reason
Aversion to company, prefers to be left alone
Fear of poverty

GENERALS:

Usually chilly, except when experiencing hot flashes

Generally worse from 3 to 5pm or 4 to 6pm

Desires chocolate, vinegary foods

Tendency toward left-sided symptoms

FEMALE HEALTH PROBLEMS:

Vaginitis, yeast infections, genital herpes

Premenstrual irritability, weepiness, and depression

Irregular timing of menses, absence of menses, or suppressed menses

Diminished libido, aversion to sex, painful sex caused by vaginal dryness

Infertility, tendency to miscarriage

Nausea of pregnancy

MODALITIES:

Generally worse from or triggered by hormonal influences (puberty, pre-menses, menses, menopause, birth control pills, pregnancy, miscarriage, etc.)

Worse from 3 to 5pm or 4 to 6pm

Ameliorated by vigorous exercise

Feels better when occupied, at work

Better from dancing

Better during thunderstorms

RELATIONSHIPS:

Complementary to *Natrum muriaticum, Nux vomica, Sabadilla*

Compare to *Natrum muriaticum, Pulsatilla, Phosphoricum acidum, Carcinosinum*

This remedy has very broad applicability. I have seen it help many women whose health problems can be traced to birth control pills, which, unbeknown to most, are capable of inducing many of the above listed symptoms. I have also seen it change the lives of a good number of women who were on the verge of leaving their marriages. They come to me complaining of, among other things, depression and unhappiness with their husband, their children, and their marriages. After a few doses of *Sepia*, their entire perspective changes for the better. This should not be interpreted as a sexist statement. While I understand that some marriages fail for very good reasons, many others can be helped, especially when the difficulties stem from a hormonal imbalance that can be corrected by this homeopathic medicine.

Without our two most important tools, the *repertory* and *materia medica*, homeopathic prescribers would be at a significant disadvantage. These references serve to organize and condense vast volumes of information into a much more manageable format. Without them, accurate prescribing would become a near impossibility. And with the advent of computer technology and its ability to make searches for specific types of information that much easier, the modern homeopath's tools have become a good bit more user friendly.

CHAPTER 5

How to Explain Homeopathy? Let Me Count the Ways...

> *The law of cure, similia similibus curentur, is as fundamental as any law in nature. It is a law of universal adaptability to human sickness; ... This is the only general law for the cure of the physical and mental ills of man; it is the only method of healing that depends, as a whole, upon one general principle, and it is the only method of healing that has continued to withstand the pressure of time and changing circumstances.*
>
> –Herbert A. Roberts, MD (1936)

When I first encountered homeopathy I was both fascinated and puzzled. I asked questions, grilled my mentors, and read books, all in search of some explanation that would satisfy my need to know. How is it possible that homeopathy can do what it appears to do? How can one or two tiny little pills yield such powerful results? What is the scientific explanation for this remarkable phenomenon that few people seem to know about? Why is there such a lack of interest on the part of the medical profession toward a therapeutic system that could revolutionize health care?

It soon became clear that of the thousands of books written on the topic dating as far back as two hundred years, very few devoted space to the issue of how or why homeopathy worked. It was as if there was an unspoken consensus that there were no answers to these questions. Even if there were, pursuing those answers was believed to be a relative waste of time, since most practitioners understood that their energies were better spent studying and practicing the homeopathic art and science of treating sick patients.

I caught on pretty quickly. I, too, became preoccupied with the nuts and bolts of practice, leaving the explanations to philosophers and scientists. The more I saw the profound impact that homeopathy could have on people's lives, the less concerned I became about needing an explanation. When trying to describe homeopathy to friends and colleagues, they would naturally respond with questions about how it worked. I was not able to answer those questions. I could only answer that it *did* work.

I knew there was not likely to ever be an explanation that would satisfy the requirements of those who see the world in conventional reductionistic, materialistic, or mechanistic terms. Intuitively, I understood that the only satisfactory answers came in the form of metaphor and, while that was sufficient for some, metaphorical answers were certainly not the type of answers that would please physicians, scientists, or skeptics.

Explanations as to how homeopathy works have no bearing on the practice of homeopathy. Now, this is not meant as a knock against all the chemists, physicists, alchemists, and poets out there trying to discover why it works. Some of them have proposed some pretty interesting theories and, I say, more power to them. For me, personally, I grew weary of wracking my brain over these issues a long time ago. I am perfectly content admitting that I don't have the foggiest notion of how or why homeopathy works. As far as I am concerned, it remains one of the great mysteries of life, and is likely to remain so for a long time to come. Physician and historian, Wilhelm Ameke, reminds us that although Hahnemann did offer hypothetical explanations for the phenomena he observed, those explanations mattered little to him. Nuts and bolts and concrete results remained his focus throughout his career.

> As the allopaths find a peculiar pleasure in refuting certain absurdities and theories of Hahnemann by the aid of our present

> knowledge, we must repeat that Hahnemann considered his theoretical explanations of no importance for his therapeutic rule. He says: "I can only vouch for the what, not for the how."[33]

Of course, this is precisely what gets scientific fundamentalists in a tizzy. They simply can't stand that homeopathy cannot be explained in conventional medical terms. Why, homeopathy defies the laws of biology, chemistry, and physics, they say. Therefore, it's just not possible. But such a conclusion requires an enormous leap of faith, which is the belief that biology, chemistry, and physics are complete sciences that already know all that can be known. The absurdity of such a notion should be readily apparent. It also represents a disingenuous double standard because there are a multitude of conventional medical principles and practices that also have no scientifically verifiable explanations. Even though the mechanisms of action of many cholesterol drugs, psychiatric medications, and even acetaminophen (Tylenol) are still unknown, no one is demanding that physicians be prohibited from prescribing them.

Although we can't say for sure how homeopathy works, there are a number of very interesting theories, many of which are quite plausible. Furthermore, no one explanation necessarily rules out all others. It is quite possible that each proposed explanation carries a kernel of truth since each one attempts to explain homeopathy from its own distinct perspective. Granted, some explanations are just descriptions of homeopathy, but this is also true of almost all conventional medical explanations. Doctors don't really know why people get asthma, for example, but they can describe mechanisms of action that produce the symptoms of asthma.

Given the confusing, controversial, and esoteric nature of the topic, I always try to tailor my explanations of homeopathy based upon my sense of the person I am addressing and the type of answers he or she will resonate with most. Although all such explanations fall short of the conventional scientific mark, they do, nevertheless, give one a sense of the uniqueness of the homeopathic perspective regarding illness and its treatment.

Homeopathy cannot be judged by conventional scientific standards because it operates from within a completely different scientific paradigm. Although these explanations are speculative, they represent legitimate attempts to conceptualize something that we don't truly understand. The following represent just a few such explanations.

Homeopathy is the science of similars

Homeopathy is the science of understanding how substances in nature can be used to treat illness based upon the similarity between the symptoms that they can cause and the symptom patterns of sick individuals. This is the straightforward explanation originally formulated by Dr. Hahnemann. It's really more a phenomenological description of the methodology. True to Hahnemann's philosophy, he described homeopathy in its most fundamental terms without offering explanations, which he believed were merely speculative and could lead to misunderstandings. Hahnemann coined the phrase, *similia similibus curentur*, or let likes be used to cure likes, to summarize the homeopathic approach.

Note that effective treatment is based upon similarity between substance and symptoms, not identicality. There is a branch of homeopathy called isopathy, which employs substances identical to the original cause (if an original cause can be identified) of an illness. An isopathic treatment for poison ivy would be *Rhus toxicodendron*, which is poison ivy in potentized homeopathic form. An illness triggered by a particular vaccine would be treated with a homeopathic dose of that vaccine. Likewise, isopathic treatment for an illness following a spider bite would involve homeopathic doses of the particular spider or spider venom in question.

There is a general consensus that homeopathy tends to be more effective when it uses similars as opposed to identicals. Which is not to say that identicals can't be useful in certain situations. It's just that similars seem to work better. It's as if the vital force responds more vigorously when faced with a stimulus slightly different from but mostly similar to the illness that it is currently grappling with.

In the case of poison ivy, therefore, substances other than poison ivy that are capable of producing itching and blistering can come in handy. In the event of a spider bite, one might get better results using a remedy made from a different spider than the one that inflicted the wound. *Apis mellifica*, a commonly used homeopathic medicine made from the honey-bee, can be useful for all sorts of bites, including spider, wasp, mosquito, tick, and even snake bites.

Homeopathy is the science of the paradoxical effect

This slightly different way of referring to Hahnemann's "law of similars" may be better received when addressing persons of a scientific bent. To such persons, I refer to homeopathy as the science of the paradoxical effect. It's really the same thing as the science of similars, just dressed up in more sophisticated language. The principle of similars becomes more comprehensible when compared to conventional medical practices that, paradoxically, defy our common understanding of how things work. Allergy shots, vaccines, and central nervous system stimulants used to treat hyperactive children are just a few such examples. Like homeopathy, these examples run counter to everyday logic. They are treatments that achieve results opposite to the effects that one might normally expect.

It should be noted that, for a number of important reasons, these conventional medical paradoxes cannot be equated with homeopathy. For one, the quantities of medicines administered are completely different. They are much larger. Furthermore, vaccines are administered across the board to all persons without regard for individual circumstances. The same is true of psychiatric treatment of attention deficit hyperactivity disorder. In both cases, the homeopathic principle of individualized prescribing is violated. A one-size-fits-all approach is anathema to homeopathic philosophy and practice.

In reality, the principle of similars is everywhere.[34] We just don't take the time to make mental note of such phenomena. When a dog eats grass, for example, in order to induce vomiting to relieve symptoms related to a digestive disturbance, it is instinctively making use of the paradoxical principle of similars. Lots of people swear by the application of an irritating substance like vinegar to alleviate the discomfort of an insect bite. Likewise, some subscribe to "a hair of the dog that bit you" the morning after in order to cut the edge off of a hangover. Folk remedies of this nature work for a real reason. In the hands of a trained homeopathic practitioner, the paradoxical principle of similars becomes a powerful tool for healing serious illness.

Homeopathy is a stimulus-response approach to healing

Another explanation that can appeal to the scientific mind is that homeopathy is based on a stimulus-response model of therapeutic intervention. Unlike conventional drugs, which are usually taken on a daily basis in order to sustain their effects, a homeopathic medicine is designed to provoke a reaction from the life force. Remedies act as catalysts that rouse the innate healing power of individual. In this stimulus-response model of therapeutics, a few doses or even a single dose may be sufficient to initiate a healing reaction. After that, the real work is done by the vital force itself.

After taking a remedy, the patient's job is to observe and report any changes that take place and to refrain from anything that might interfere with those changes (such as coffee, drugs, etc.). The job of the practitioner is to evaluate those changes in order to determine whether the vital force is responding in an effective manner. If there is no response or the response is not productive, the practitioner chooses a different remedy to stimulate the life force. If the response is positive but then begins to wear off, the practitioner may choose to repeat the stimulus.

Now, compare this to the fact that many conventional drugs must be taken on an indefinite basis. Otherwise, their effects can quickly wear off. Stop that blood pressure medication and one's blood pressure is likely to rise again. Discontinue that anti-inflammatory drug and one's arthritic pain is likely to return in short order. This illustrates the point that almost all drugs act in a suppressive manner, keeping symptoms temporarily at bay. In many cases, the life force eventually rebels, either by intensifying the illness, or by expressing itself in new ways through new symptoms and new illnesses. In the first instance, higher doses of medicine and, sometimes, additional medicines are needed to keep the same symptoms under control. In the latter case, conventional medicine almost uniformly fails to acknowledge the connection between its suppressive treatments and the new illnesses that they engender.

The two approaches—allopathic and homeopathic—represent a quantum difference in understanding regarding the nature of the vital energy and how it responds to various therapeutic interventions. One method aims to counteract the efforts of the life force to heal itself, while the other seeks to work in concert with the self-healing capacity of the organism. One unwittingly chooses suppression as its primary mode of action, while homeopathy consciously and deliberately takes advantage of the innate healing capacity of the vital life energy. The long-term outcomes are profoundly different. One perpetuates the inevitability of chronic disease, while the other promotes genuine healing.

Homeopathy is an energy medicine that restores the bioenergetic life force to balance

This particular explanation can appeal to those who are a bit more open-minded and willing to think outside the box. I like to explain to such persons that conventional medicine operates at the levels of biology and chemistry. Drugs intervene on a biochemical level seeking to alter specific biochemical pathways and physiological processes. Surgeries intervene on an anatomical level, oftentimes removing organs or parts of organs that are believed to be irreversibly diseased. In the old days, tonsils were favorite targets of surgeons; nowadays we routinely remove gallbladders, appendixes, and prostates when they cause too much trouble.

In addition to biology and chemistry, medicine also makes use of physics, but mostly in terms of diagnostics and rarely as a form of therapeutics. Ultrasound, thermography, magnetic resonance imaging (MRI), computed tomography (CT scans), and good old-fashioned X-rays are all technologies that could not have been developed without science's understanding of physics. Such technologies, in my opinion, are one of the great strengths of conventional medicine.

However, when conventional medicine employs its knowledge of physics to develop treatments, they turn out to be rather destructive. We all know how damaging radiation therapy for cancer can be for both the cancer and the patient. Radioactive iodine therapy is administered with the intention of destroying a dysfunctional thyroid gland that has run amok. It is understood that after the thyroid has been obliterated, the patient will need hormone replacement therapy, which comes in the form of a variety of thyroid hormone analogs.

Conventional medicine's shortcoming is that it fails to apply physics in a constructive manner to therapeutics. Fortunately, this is where homeopathy excels. Homeopathy is based on the application of physics to medical therapeutics. This is why it is referred to as a form of energy medicine. It may not use energy in a way that is comprehensible to conventional physics, but it clearly operates at the level of subtle energy exemplified and manifested by the life force itself.

Even conventional science acknowledges the existence of electromagnetic fields in relation to life forms. Skeptics scoff at the notion, but there are some sensitive individuals who can visualize the auras that surround human beings. The human aura is just another way of referring to the electromagnetic field or bioenergetic life force that surrounds, permeates, and charges the living organism. Homeopathy has developed a therapeutic science that makes use of subtle energies designed to intervene at the level of the bioenergetic life force.

The phenomenon of constructive interference is a basic tenet of classical physics. When two energy waves with similar characteristics come together, they can reinforce each other and combine to form a more powerful energy wave. Applied to homeopathic healing, we can say that the life force of a sick individual vibrates in a manner out of character from its normal healthy state. It is said to be out of balance.

The homeopath seeks a substance from nature that vibrates at a similar frequency to the out-of-sync vital force. This is accomplished by matching up the symptom profiles of the two.

An out of balance life force is recognized by the specific symptoms that it generates. In fact, those symptoms represent the life force's attempt to heal itself. But sometimes it needs a little assistance. The energy signature of a given substance is recognized by the symptoms that it can cause when taken by a healthy person. The energy of the substance in the form of a homeopathically prepared medicine is chosen with the intention of matching the out-of-balance energy of the sick individual.

The similar energies are brought together by administering doses of the homeopathic medicine to the sick person. If the energies are similar enough to each other, they vibrate in such a way as to create a therapeutic form of constructive interference. In other words, when the two frequencies resonate sufficiently, it triggers a healing response. The original but failed attempt of the vital force to heal itself is reinforced, thus generating a stronger energy capable of overcoming the state of imbalance represented by the illness, thereby restoring the sick person to health.

Basic science teaches that without chemistry there could be no biology. It is also true that without physics there could be no chemistry. The forces described by physics drive all material forces in the universe including human biology, chemistry, and physiology. Surgical removal of a body part, therefore, is the crudest and least effective form of therapeutic intervention because the scope of its impact is relatively limited. Note that this is not to say that surgery is never advisable. Sometimes it is the wisest course of action.

Chemical interventions in the form of drug therapies are less crude and have the potential to generate a wider influence on the organism, both in positive and negative ways. Energetic interventions like homeopathy and some other forms of energy medicine operate at the level of physics, or perhaps at the level of an even more sophisticated form of subtle energy, a type of energy that physics has yet to acknowledge.

Interventions at the level of subtle energy have the capacity to alter the human organism in an all-encompassing manner that affects the entire organism. Therapeutic interventions at the energetic level can influence both chemistry and biology in profound ways.

Homeopathy releases the life force from the negative feedback loop of illness

This explanation builds upon the prior one, using metaphorical language that paints a picture of the physics of the organism in its healthy and unhealthy states. According to this explanation, we can conceptualize illness as a dysfunctional negative feedback loop that holds the life force in place, rendering it unable to respond in a healthy manner to stressors that impinge upon the organism. At some point in time, a negative influence or influences threw the healthy vital force out of sync. It remained out of balance, stuck in a new holding pattern, unable to return to its previous healthy state of balance. As a consequence, the life force repeatedly or continuously generates the same symptom pattern, a sign that it is unable to break free from the influence of a negative energetic feedback loop.

Symptoms that do not resolve through the efforts of the vital force are the symptoms of chronic illness. All chronic illness can be seen as a function of a life force that is unable to heal itself, unable to restore homeostasis. The life force will likely remain stuck in this dysfunctional energy vortex until an additional negative influence pushes it further into a deeper state of pathological dysfunction or until a strong enough positive influence jars it back to its previous state of health and balance.

Remember, too, that the symptom pattern generated by the vital force represents its best effort to heal itself. When this self-healing mechanism fails, it bogs down and remains stuck, thus repeating the same symptom pattern indefinitely. Realizing that this specific symptom pattern is a failed effort of the life force to heal itself, homeopathy seeks to bolster that effort in the hope of releasing the life force from the grip of the vortex. This is accomplished by selecting a substance in nature that is capable of causing very similar symptoms. A potentized medicine that matches the symptom profile of the illness, and is designed to mimic the efforts of the life force, can act to jar the stuck vital energy loose from its negative feedback loop. The life force is thus freed from the vortex and able to return to a more resilient and balanced state. It becomes capable once again of responding in an effective manner to any further negative influences.

Homeopathy is constitutional medicine

A popular and appealing way to explain homeopathy, one that differentiates it from mainstream approaches to health, is to refer to it as *constitutional medicine*. This immediately conveys the idea that homeopathic treatment involves more than just symptomatic relief. The constitution consists of the spiritual, mental, emotional, and physical makeup of the whole person. The health, strength, and vitality of the underlying constitution are the most important factors in healing. A weak constitution is going to have a hard time handling adverse circumstances and recovering from illness.

The aim of homeopathy is to strengthen the underlying constitution, thus enabling it to ward off illness and restore the sick person to health. A homeopathic practitioner studies the overall symptom pattern of the sick individual in order to understand his or her constitutional makeup. A homeopathic medicine chosen on this basis is designed to heal the whole person, not just a specific symptom or set of symptoms. This is what is meant by the term, *constitutional prescribing*.

This, of course, is a drastic departure from the haphazard way in which conventional medicine seeks to indiscriminately extinguish individual symptoms without regard for their purpose or overall role in the maintenance of health of the organism. Such an approach is usually at odds with the innate wisdom of the vital force, which is why conventional drugs are so prone to generating side effects. Contrary to what the term suggests, *side effects* are not simply minor peripheral effects that accompany the beneficial effects of drugs. They are, in actuality, the direct effects of drugs. Not only that, but side effects have the same origin as all other symptoms; they represent protest signals produced by an unhappy and disordered vital force.

Once again, if symptoms are understood to be the life force's best efforts to heal itself, one has to seriously reconsider a medical strategy the sole purpose of which is to wage war against any and all symptoms. It only follows that such a strategy, while admittedly capable of producing temporary symptomatic relief, would also have a distinct tendency to undermine the constitutional health of the individual. Orthodox medicine takes a short-term approach that focuses on individual symptoms and artificial diagnostic labels, neither of which are sufficiently representative of the underlying constitution. Homeopathy takes a longer view. It is purposely designed to heal the whole by reinforcing the defenses of the constitution.

Homeopathy is the medical science of ultra-low dose therapeutics

This pharmacological interpretation of the mechanism of action of homeopathic medicines should be of interest to any scientific-minded person. Homeopathic doses are extremely dilute. No homeopath denies this. And yet the medicines made by the process of serial dilution and succussion still seem to work. In fact, homeopathic clinicians have observed that they work far better than stronger, cruder doses of the same substances.

Dr. Hahnemann was the first to discover an actual method by which to produce and apply ultra-low doses of medicines. A proposed scientific explanation for this phenomenon came later in the nineteenth century in the form of the Arndt-Schulz principle.[35] Dr. Rudolph Arndt, a psychiatrist, and Hugo Schulz, a pharmacologist, were early pioneers in the field of pharmacology. Together, their investigations led to an understanding of the dose-dependent effect of medicines, which is to say that a given substance can produce widely different results depending upon the quantity administered.

Schulz' experiments revealed that different doses of various substances could either stimulate or inhibit the growth of yeast. Interestingly, around the same time period, Dr. Ferdinand Hueppe observed a similar phenomenon regarding the inhibition and stimulation of growth in bacteria. In short, the Arndt-Schulz principle states that high concentrations of certain substances create a destructive effect, medium concentrations have an inhibitory effect, and low concentrations produce a stimulatory effect. Put in different terms, strong stimuli can have a toxic effect on physiologic processes, medium strength stimuli can inhibit physiology, and weak stimuli can actually serve to enhance physiologic activity.

The Arndt-Schulz principle demonstrates the differences between crude conventional pharmacological drug doses, which are employed mainly to suppress symptoms and are known to produce a variety of harmful side effects, and highly diluted homeopathic medicines, which are designed to stimulate and encourage the self-healing capacity of the life force and come with a minimum of side effects. Antibiotics, for example, must be given in sufficient quantity to either inhibit or kill targeted bacteria. In contrast, homeopathic doses stimulate the immune system to rouse its defenses against bacterial colonization.

The Arndt-Schulz principle was a mainstay of pharmacological theory for decades. It was later replaced by the modern scientific discipline called *hormesis*. Although hormesis attributes its origins to Hugo Schulz, the term was originally coined in a scientific paper published by C.M. Southam and J. Ehrlich in 1943 after they were surprised to discover that low concentrations of an antibiotic had an effect opposite to what they had anticipated—it stimulated the growth of a fungus.[36]

Nowadays, hormesis is a term used in toxicology to refer to the study of a biphasic dose phenomenon characterized by the inhibitory effects caused by high or toxic doses of substances versus the stimulatory impact of low doses. Although it is not well recognized, hormesis is fast becoming a serious scientific discipline with a growing body of research. There are now scientific journals and professional societies devoted to the topic.

The great irony is that Hahnemann and his healing art of homeopathy are rarely given the credit that they deserve. Any way you slice it, whether we call it hormesis or the Arndt-Schulz principle, Hahnemann had applied this little-known phenomenon to the art and science of healing well before its supposed scientific namesakes had described it decades later. Whether acknowledged by mainstream science or not, homeopathy *is* the hormetic science of low dose medicinal effects. Homeopathy studies the effects of high, medium, and low doses of substances and, based upon that information, prescribes ultra-low doses to catalyze healing responses in sick individuals.

Homeopathy heals with complex dilutions that contain energetic imprints of medicinal substances

In 1988, Dr. Jacques Benveniste ignited a firestorm of controversy in the scientific world when he published an article in the journal, *Nature*.[37] In that paper, he noted that he had observed a rather strange phenomenon. His research suggested that an antigen could still provoke an immune response from white blood cells even after the antigen had been diluted in water to the point at which there was no longer any of the antigen left in solution. The solution had been prepared in the same manner as a homeopathic medicine, through a step-wise process of dilution and vigorous shaking.

Benveniste, a physician and research director at the French National Institute for Medical Research, who is also renowned for his 1971 discovery of *platelet activating factor*, theorized that the process of dilution and succussion had resulted in a transfer of biological information from the original antigen to the remaining water solution. Later, in a magazine interview, Benveniste described his groundbreaking discovery:

> *It's known as the "memory of water." When you add a substance to water and then dilute the water to the point where there are no more molecules of the added substance left in the water, you can still measure effects of the water as if the originally diluted substance were still present.*[38]

In spite of corroborating evidence produced by three additional labs that replicated his research, *Nature* later published a refutation of

Benveniste's work written by a team of "debunkers." That team included the editor of *Nature* himself, John Maddox, and infamous magician and anti-holistic medicine crusader, James Randi. Talk about conflict of interest and bias! The very word, debunker, oozes with bias. Knowing that Benveniste's research might confirm what homeopaths across the globe have known for two hundred years, they had set out to ensure that it would not happen. As a consequence, Benveniste's research funding was withdrawn and his reputation within the mainstream scientific community was irreparably damaged.

Nevertheless, Benveniste's ideas regarding the memory of water have sparked a great deal of interest and subsequent research. In 2010, Luc Montagnier, a French virologist who was awarded a Nobel Prize for his work in helping discover the *human immunodeficiency virus* (HIV), added fuel to the fire during an interview with *Science* magazine when he remarked:

> *I can't say that homeopathy is right in everything. What I can say now is that the high dilutions are right. High dilutions of something are not nothing. They are water structures which mimic the original molecules.*[39]

He had come to this conclusion as a result of his research involving high dilutions of DNA, the results of which were published in 2009.

> *What we have found is that DNA produces structural changes in water, which persists at very high dilutions, and which lead to resonant electromagnetic signals that we can measure.*[40]

Faced with a similar firestorm of scientific intolerance, Montagnier discussed his future plans during the *Science* interview. He spoke of Jacques Benveniste as "a modern Galileo," a reference to the Italian scientist who had famously endured religious persecution for his heretical ideas during the Renaissance. When asked if his research interests constituted "pseudoscience," Montagnier revealed that he had decided to leave Paris in order to pursue his work at Jiaotong University in

China where he hoped to avoid the "intellectual terror" that innovative thinkers tend to encounter in mainstream Western scientific academic circles.

Well-known English author and biologist, Rupert Sheldrake, has met with similar resistance from the mainstream scientific community for his theory of *morphic resonance*, which, by the way, is remarkably compatible with the memory of water concept embodied by homeopathic dilutions. Sheldrake believes that "memory is inherent in nature" and that natural systems such as plants, animals, and even molecules "inherit a collective memory from all previous things of their kind."

To illustrate the pervasive nature of opposition to new ideas within mainstream science, here is what *Wikipedia*—that safe haven for homeopathy haters, skeptics, and scientific fundamentalists that poses as a bastion of legitimate science—has to say about Sheldrake and his theory:

> *Morphic resonance is not accepted by the scientific community as a real phenomenon and Sheldrake's proposals relating to it have been characterized as pseudoscience. Critics cite a lack of evidence for morphic resonance and an inconsistency of the idea with data from genetics and embryology, and also express concern that popular attention from Sheldrake's books and public appearances undermines the public's understanding of science.*[41]

Suffice it to say, a growing preponderance of evidence supported by cutting-edge science points to the fact that homeopathic high dilutions are capable of stimulating biological activity, even when the material doses involved are miniscule to non-existent. All homeopaths know this and, when patients receiving homeopathic care experience relief from their chronic ailments, they know it too.

Although we can only speculate regarding the exact mechanism by which information is transferred from solute to solvent in homeopathic dilutions, the fact is that something profound and paradigm shattering does occur. The bottom line is that the process of serial dilution and succussion seems to leave an energetic imprint of the original medicinal substance on the remaining highly dilute homeopathic solution. That energy can be harnessed in such a way as to maximize its therapeutic benefits while minimizing the side effects that would normally be expected from the crude undiluted substance.

Homeopathy is the art and science of nanopharmacological medicine

This particular line of thinking can be especially appealing to those who refuse to accept explanations based in bioenergetics. Such persons require an explanation involving a material mechanism in order to accept the possibility that homeopathic medicines are not just placebos. Researchers have discovered that, contrary to what science formerly assumed, homeopathic dilutions do contain tiny amounts of original substance. It was previously believed that dilution of a substance beyond a certain point would result in a solution that is unlikely to contain even a single molecule of that original substance.

The laws of chemistry reveal that this point, the limit beyond which one can dilute a substance thereby rendering it unlikely that even a single molecule will remain, corresponds to what is known as Avogadro's number. This endpoint of dilution is mathematically represented by the number 6.023×10^{23}. For example, basic math tells us that a common homeopathic potency known as 12C is diluted to the point where the final solution contains one part per 10^{24} parts. This level of dilution is beyond the factor represented by Avogadro's number. Skeptics like to harp on this concept because they believe that it provides evidence proving that it is impossible for homeopathy to work, since it presumably violates the laws of chemistry.

Of course, this controversy has swirled around homeopathy since the time of Hahnemann. Skeptics hang their entire argument on the idea that homeopathic doses are too miniscule to have any appreciable chemical, biological, or physiological effect. Most skeptics are unwilling to admit that the actions of homeopathic medicines could have any scientific basis. And much of mainstream science has been in agreement with the skeptics—until just recently.

In 2010, researchers in India unexpectedly discovered nanoparticles in the solutions produced by the homeopathic potentization process:

> ...we have demonstrated for the first time by Transmission Electron Microscopy (TEM), electron diffraction and chemical analysis by Inductively Coupled Plasma-Atomic Emission Spectroscopy (ICP-AES), the presence of physical entities in these extreme dilutions, in the form of nanoparticles of the starting metals and their aggregates.[42]

In 2012, researchers from the University of Arizona College of Medicine published a paper proposing a mechanism of action by which homeopathically prepared nanoparticles might exert their influence. They concluded that:

> The proposed model suggests that homeopathy is not only scientifically "plausible," but also grounded in an extensive empirical research literature. Homeopathic remedies come into existence and exert their biological effects mainly as nanostructures... The resultant findings on what homeopathic remedies are (highly reactive nanoparticles) and how they interact with complex living systems (as pulsed, low level doses of a salient and novel environmental stressor) could significantly advance the field as a valuable form of nanomedicine.[43]

The research division of the American Medical College of Homeopathy offered this explanation regarding the nature of nanopharmacological microdoses and their potential effects:

> Nanoparticle forms of natural medicinal agents such as herbs and minerals and of conventional synthetic drugs have enhanced biological effects, usually leading to lower doses separated in time from one another, longer durations of action, better targeting, and fewer side effects. Because of their small size and associated re-

> *active surfaces, tiny concentrations of certain nanoparticles even down to the parts per billion range are still very active chemically and biologically... Nanochemists and nanotoxicologists have discovered that smaller particles and more dilute solutions are sometimes more powerful chemically and biologically than more concentrated solutions of nanoparticles.*[44]

The implication of this recent trend in research is that homeopathic dilutions do actually contain tiny particles or microdoses of medicines that are capable of triggering changes in biological systems. In other words, according to this explanation, Hahnemann pioneered the field of nanopharmacological medicine over two hundred years ago. And modern science is just now catching up with his remarkable discoveries. But as we have seen, Hahnemann wasn't concerned with explanations. He believed his time was better spent on the actual treatment of patients.

As expected, skeptics howl in protest at the notion of homeopathic nanopharmacology because they are not interested in the actual science as much as they are intent on defaming the name of homeopathy. Nevertheless, the debate rages on and a whole new field of medical research has been birthed.

In my opinion, although this does represent a deeper level explanation of the effects observed by homeopathic practitioners and their patients, it is not the final answer. It represents just another material explanation for a much more complex phenomenon that I believe will never be able to be understood in purely material terms. I commend the researchers and wish them well, but I believe any final answer to the riddle of homeopathy—if that is even possible—lies beyond the bounds of conventional materialist science. Short of a final answer, the homeopathy as nanomedicine theory remains the best answer to those who insist that homeopathic medicines cannot work because they consist of nothing but water.

Homeopathy is true mind-body medicine in its most complete form

Conventional medicine acknowledges the power of the mind to create illness but then invariably resorts to material interventions for all health problems whether of mind or body. Medicine provides pills for every type of sneeze, sniffle, ache, and pain. And there are lots more pills for depression, anxiety, overactive minds, and just about any other kind of mental and emotional problem that one can imagine. Material doses of crude and oftentimes dangerous drugs have become the standard short-term answer to all our worldly woes.

There is a pervasive stigma regarding mental and emotional health issues. Few hesitate to tell friends of their visits to the doctor, while many hide the truth about their having seen a therapist or psychiatrist. We fail to take the psyche seriously, deluding ourselves into believing that it is possible to get to the root of things through biochemical means. We have been led to believe that scientific investigation of the physical brain can somehow unlock the secrets of the mind. Our materialist bias and fear of looking too closely at our inner selves guarantee that the trend will continue. As a consequence, mental illness and human suffering continue to increase in spite of the best efforts of our state-of-the-art medical system.

Now let's compare this to the homeopathic perspective. To a homeopath, feelings of self-loathing, jealousy, or lack of confidence are no different than symptoms like heartburn, joint aches, or diarrhea. They all represent signs of a disordered vital force. They are clues that point to a potential solution. During an interview, I often swing back and forth, asking questions first about a person's asthma, then about his sleep patterns, his food cravings, his anger issues, his fears, and then back again to physical concerns like his stiff back and itchy eyes. This is perhaps the thing I love most about homeopathy. I must simultaneously think like a general practitioner and a psychiatrist. As far as the homeopath is concerned, there is no division between mind and body.

To me, it's all one. It's all the same. There is no judgment. I talk about the color of the mucus a person blows from her nose with the same tone and demeanor that I discuss the social inadequacy that she experiences while attending business conventions. The patient comes away from the homeopathic interview with the impression that all information, whether of a physical or emotional nature, is potentially valuable to the prescriber, and that he or she will not be judged when revealing that information. The ultimate goal is to find medicines that match the overall symptom patterns of patients, not to pigeonhole them with psychiatric labels that make them feel bad about themselves. The net effect is to diminish the stigma that people with psychological difficulties can be made to feel.

Homeopaths know that mental/emotional symptoms are on a par with physical symptoms. They simply represent clues to the sleuthing homeopath who is searching for a remedy that will match the symptom profile of the suffering individual. Most telling of all is the fact that I have seen cases of physical pathology solved by virtue of psychological clues, and I have chosen correct remedies for emotional problems based on physical clues.

Let's use the example of a man seeking help for chronic hives. Careful questioning reveals that the hives began shortly after the death of a parent, and that he has a tendency to internalize his grief. He acknowledges being unable to cry. Most homeopaths would concur that this is a pretty straightforward case and would also agree on the choice of remedy for this man's hives. Most would also expect that even though the patient sought help for hives, the remedy should also act to unblock his grief. Since they are not separate concerns, both the hives and grief should resolve if the correct homeopathic medicine is given. (Remedy choice?[45])

Another patient presents with a chief complaint of depression ever since adolescence. Questioning reveals that she has had two miscarriages, she feels best when she exercises, feels tired from 3 to 5pm, has a strong desire for chocolate, and can get headaches that center above her left eye. Any good homeopathic practitioner immediately knows the indicated remedy in such a case. It is reasonable to expect that the correct remedy will not only eliminate the depression; it will also resolve the headaches, diminish the chocolate craving, give her more energy in the afternoons, and reduce the likelihood of another miscarriage. (Remedy choice?[46])

Just to be clear, it is also possible that the solution to a physical health problem can be found by virtue of additional physical clues. A case of abdominal cramps may be quickly resolved when it is revealed that the pain is temporarily relieved by firm pressure, warm applications, and bringing the knees up to the abdomen. (Remedy choice?[47])

Likewise, it is possible to solve emotional problems through the use of emotional clues. The remedy choice for a man with anger problems becomes apparent when he acknowledges that he has a strong streak of jealousy that causes him to imagine that his wife's innocent conversations with other men are a threat to his marriage. The observant homeopath notes that this man is quite talkative. He also admits to having a fear of snakes. (Remedy choice?[48])

There is no greater testament to the absolute unity of mind and body than the clinical results produced by homeopathic treatment. Mind and body are not just intimately connected; they are one and the same. Homeopaths understand this and use that knowledge to achieve powerful results. No other healing modality is capable of producing such results with the same degree of consistency.

In this sense, homeopathy defies the conventional medical paradigm, which, at best, sees mind and body as separate entities and, at worst, ignores the psyche while focusing solely on the physical body in search of material solutions. One can only conclude that homeopathic healing is a very unusual phenomenon, one that transcends the boundaries of materialist medical science.

Mind and body are one and must be treated as one. When they are treated separately, as is the case with conventional medicine, the results are often superficial, short-lived, and fraught with unforeseen difficulties. When a patient says, "I know that my stomach pains are caused by my anxiety about the health of my child," the homeopath trusts this to be a potentially valuable piece of information. Homeopathy passes no judgment, excludes no information, and takes patient's reports of their own experiences at face value. The success of homeopathy rests on this critical understanding of mind and body as two inseparable aspects of the same whole.

Homeopathy is the final realization and practical application of the ancient science of alchemy

This explanation is my personal favorite because it encompasses the tremendous potential of homeopathy in its broadest terms. It will not likely appeal to those who require scientific certainty, but it will pique the interest of many who are willing to think beyond the boundaries of conventional science. I devoted a chapter to this explanation in my book, *Green Medicine*,[49] so I won't go into as much depth on the topic here.

Alchemy, like astrology, is sneered at by skeptics who believe it to be unscientific claptrap. In truth, alchemy was the ancient precursor to modern day chemistry. As such, it deserves a great deal more respect than it receives. Skeptics miss the point entirely when they dismiss alchemy as naïve. They fail to understand that alchemy was not intended to be a purely material science. Its purpose was not to synthesize new molecular entities and chemical compounds. Its aims were much higher.

Alchemy was a spiritual-chemical discipline that sought to transform human consciousness through methods that were symbolically represented by the activities of alchemists in their alchemical laboratories. Alchemists famously sought to transmute the base metal, lead, into the most precious of all metals, gold. The alchemist's "outer" work in the laboratory was a reflection of and complement to the "inner" work of initiation, individuation, and transformation taking place in the soul/psyche of the alchemist. While these pioneers of chemistry developed a variety of practical laboratory techniques along the way on their quest for the mythical philosopher's stone, their true agenda was inner psychological and spiritual growth.

Chemistry is the modern-day materially oriented scientific cousin of ancient alchemy, stripped of all the symbolic meaning and significance that alchemy once held. The crossroads where chemistry diverges from alchemy is the same place where skeptics and more open-minded thinkers part ways. Skeptics are scientific purists who are interested only in the strict material aspects of science. Seekers, healers, and patients in need of healing, on the other hand, understand that there is a great deal more to healing than can be encompassed by profane science.

The alchemists were involved in an epic quest, searching for the secrets that would unlock the spiritual power of matter, that could transmute everyday lead into pure gold. Many now understand this as a metaphor for the process by which genuine healing takes place. Herein lies the difference between homeopathic and allopathic treatment. There is nothing extraordinary about applying crude drugs to individual symptoms in order to beat them into submission. Its goal is to maintain the status quo and nothing more. However, something truly extraordinary can take place when a homeopathic remedy initiates a healing response. It often results in resolution of illness while simultaneously promoting greater awareness, emotional maturity, and psychological growth.

Homeopathic healing sounds like a very tall order—because it is. It is not something that can be accomplished with crude pharmaceuticals, the alchemical equivalent of base lead. It requires something capable of acting not just on the material plane, but also on the invisible, immaterial plane of spirit, mind, and soul. In fact, it requires something that can bridge the gap between matter and spirit, between body and mind. Homeopathy does more than just bridge the gap. It does not recognize a gap because there is no gap. All is one.

Hahnemann knew that he was onto something extraordinary when he diluted his medicines in order to minimize their side effects, only to find that their power to heal became even stronger. Without purposely setting out to do so, Hahnemann had discovered a practical method—serial dilution and succussion—by which to magnify the energetic or spiritual power of matter. He had accomplished the very thing that the alchemists had intuited long ago but were unable to achieve in the practical everyday sense. Two centuries ago, Hahnemann understood the significance of this monumental discovery:

> *The finest dose is almost nothing but pure, freely unveiled, spirit-like medicinal energy, and carries out—only dynamically—such great actions as could never be achieved by the raw medicinal substance, even when it is taken in a large dose.*[50]

It is my contention that homeopathy is the Magnum Opus, the green elixir, the philosopher's stone that the alchemists were questing after. Its power to heal is unparalleled. The creation of homeopathic medicines is analogous to the alchemical transmutation of base substances into their dynamic spiritual counterparts. And the administration of the correct remedy, the *simillimum*, has a similar power to transform body, mind, and soul.

Take the venom of the Bushmaster snake, *Lachesis mutus*, for example. In its crude form it is a dangerous cardiovascular toxin that has been known to cause fatalities. In its potentized homeopathic form, it is a broad-spectrum agent that can heal deep-seated physical and psychological problems. By virtue of Hahnemann's discovery, we now have the ability to unleash the inner healing power of any earthly substance. And when the correct medicine is matched with the corresponding totality of symptoms of the sick person, it can catalyze a transformation that is not unlike the pure gold of alchemical legend.

Additional theories

I'm sure my homeopathic colleagues have their own favorite explanations, including some that I have not mentioned. All such explanations represent legitimate attempts to describe a phenomenon that is not fully understood. Such explanations are not necessarily mutually exclusive. All explanations that I offer here may turn out to be true. One thing is for sure, though. The lack of satisfactory scientific explanation for homeopathy in no way invalidates its remarkable power to heal. Just ask anyone who has experienced it firsthand.

Cutting edge science is one of the best places to look for answers. Epigenetics is an emerging field of great scientific interest. Some claim that the answers to the mysteries of homeopathy will be found there. Theoretical physics is a particularly fruitful field in terms of investigating potential mechanisms for homeopathic medicines. Physics has already proposed more theories than I have described here. Some are too involved to discuss in a book like this and, admittedly, too complex for me to even understand.

Nevertheless, it is still my belief that science—at least conventional science as it is currently configured—is too narrow in its scope to fully grasp the extent of the homeopathic phenomenon. All scientific explanations are fated to be incomplete from the outset because they are, by definition, reductionist in nature. Holism will never be able to be understood in reductionist terms. The same applies to materialist perspectives. An immaterial phenomenon can never be explained in material terms.

Perhaps a revolution in scientific method similar to the type I have proposed in my book, *Metaphysics & Medicine*,[51] will be capable some day of explaining homeopathy, but I am not too optimistic about that prospect. Homeopathy is likely to remain a mystery for eons to come. And honestly, I don't think I mind that.

CHAPTER 6

How We Get Sick and Why

Metaphorically speaking, disease is resistance.
    –Stuart Close, MD (1924)

Any disturbance of this vital energy immediately shows itself in lack of harmony through the outward manifestations of our beings; in other words, symptoms. When harmonious functioning is disturbed, we get sickness as a result, and it has as its base and inception this lack of harmony in the flow of vital energy through the body. This is manifest in disease as it naturally develops because of disturbed vital force...
    –Herbert A. Roberts, MD (1936)

Human beings are remarkably vulnerable to all manner of deleterious influences. An adult can contract pneumonia from a draft of cold air. Waking just an hour too late can make some people suffer for the rest of the day. A grown man can sink into depression when his favorite team loses the big game. A child can be made to suffer from a disapproving glance. Is humanity really that fragile? Yes, I'm afraid that we are. While we are all susceptible to the big stressors, like the death of a loved one or the loss of a job, we are also capable of being wounded by seemingly innocuous events.

The good news is that while human beings are remarkably fragile, they are also remarkably resilient. We can withstand a great deal of trauma to both mind and body. We have the innate self-healing capacity of the life force to thank for this ability to persevere. The vital force has tremendous power to heal—and to compensate for problems that can't be healed. Since the life force does not heal all insults, the wounds that remain must be carried, sometimes over the duration of a lifetime.

The world is full of the walking wounded. Most manage to adjust to the wounds that they carry. The human race is highly adept at camouflaging suffering and compensating for its effects. The socially awkward young student compensates by overachieving in academics. The sexually traumatized woman avoids intimate relationships to maintain her psychic sense of safety. The successful businessman hides behind his wealth to make up for his inner sense of inadequacy. Nowadays, most everyone uses symptom-suppressing medications to aid in the cover-up. The average person can carry a tremendous amount of suffering while simultaneously projecting an appearance of normalcy to the outside world.

Over the years, layers of accumulated trauma and pain tend to take their toll. And, yet, most manage to keep it together, building up a protective armor of defense—until one day the damn finally bursts. In the early stages, before the damn gives way, distress signals produced by the vital force usually take the form of run-of-the-mill acute ailments like colds, headaches, and short-lived viral illnesses. But as the life force's defenses weaken, it becomes increasingly susceptible to chronic illness. This is when we begin to see conditions like arthritis, high blood pressure, depression, anxiety disorders, heart disease, and diabetes.

Fortunately, with a little patience and persistence, homeopathy has the ability to peel away the layers, to restore one's health piece by piece. While this cannot always be accomplished for all people at all times, there is nothing else that is capable of digging down that deep to restore health and vitality to so many with such consistency.

Origins of disease

The origin of disease is a highly complex topic, one that is incapable of being summarized in straightforward terms. The standard "nature versus nurture" debate, which pits genetic against environmental factors as the primary reasons for disease, is a gross oversimplification. The biases deeply ingrained in our scientific culture skew medicine's search for causes in the direction of genetic factors. This is primarily because genes are tangible, material entities that can be studied by science.

Although they may be less quantifiable, social, economic, psychological, spiritual, and environmental factors are every bit as real as genetic factors. Nevertheless, the bias of modern science predisposes it to favor material causes of disease that can be detected by its instruments and manipulated in its labs. Medicine consistently downplays the human factor, the very thing that defines what it is to be a living, breathing being. It does so because the psyche and its effects cannot be isolated in a lab for the purposes of being dissected and measured.

From a homeopathic perspective, there is much more to illness than meets the scientific eye. Broadly speaking, both constitutional and environmental factors need to be taken into account. Constitutional factors are those factors that we come into the world with. Environmental factors are all other factors that impinge upon our daily lives after we have arrived. We inherit constitutional influences and we acquire environmental influences. This may sound a lot like the nature-nurture dichotomy but it is not. Allow me to explain.

When medicine refers to the nature component of disease it is referring to genetic inheritance. Factors that are relatively hardwired into our makeup are a function of genetic inheritance. Genes determine things like our gender, hair and eye color, and body types. These are characteristics that are unlikely to ever change. Because it is a genetically hardwired condition, a child with Down syndrome will always have Down syndrome. However, there is much more to inheritance than fixed traits like our blood types.

Genetic versus energetic inheritance

While conventional medicine assumes all inherited influences to be genetic, homeopathy understands inheritance to be both *genetic* and *energetic*. In fact, the vast majority of inherited factors that influence our health are energetic, which is to say that they are not irreversibly hardwired into our constitutional makeup. Since energetic influences are not permanently encoded within our DNA, it is possible that they can be altered in our favor. Changes of this nature cannot, however, be accomplished through chemical, biological, or surgical means. Inherited energetic influences can only be changed via interventions of a similar energetic nature. Because it is a specific and comprehensive form of energy medicine, this is where homeopathy excels.

The following are a few common examples designed to illustrate what I mean by energetic inheritance.

Example 1

An adult who was physically beaten on a regular basis as a child conceives his own child who, at an early age, before most behaviors are learned, displays similar emotional traits as the father. The child acts timid, hypersensitive to angry tones of voice, and withdrawn, just like the father who attributes the same traits in himself to his having been abused as a child.

Here we have an example where the energetic imprint of the acquired emotional dysfunction of the parent is transmitted to the child. Since this transference is not genetic and it is not learned, it must be attributed to the phenomenon of energetic inheritance. This is a ubiquitous phenomenon that routinely can occur anywhere between conception and birth.

Example 2

A grieving woman who has lost both of her parents within the past three years conceives a child who cries incessantly and refuses to nurse. It turns out that the mother, too, has a tendency to cry frequently and has experienced diminished appetite since losing her parents.

This is similar to *Example 1* in that an acquired emotional state is transferred to the child. Note that in the normal process of grieving a person moves through the various stages of grief to a reasonable conclusion. In this case, the mother continues to cry frequently and lacks for appetite years after the death of her parents. This is an indication that she is "stuck" in the energetic vortex of her grief, unable to break free from its grip. When the infant displays similar symptoms we can assume that it, too, has been caught up in a similar energy vortex.

Example 3

A child with chronic respiratory problems including a history of croup, frequent coughs, bronchitis, and asthma, has a grandparent who contracted tuberculosis before conceiving his son, the father of the child with respiratory problems.

This is a well-recognized syndrome that has been observed by homeopathic doctors for almost two centuries. In this case, a tubercular influence that originates in a grandparent who had tuberculosis is energetically transferred down through the generations. Its effect is to create a predisposition toward respiratory problems (among other things) in those affected by this "miasm." In homeopathy, the word *miasm* is used to denote a predisposition toward certain types of symptoms and illnesses. The term is used by some to refer more specifically to the energetic influence of infectious agents upon one's constitutional health. Miasmatic theory is a complex and sometimes controversial topic within homeopathic circles.

The bottom line is that there is a homeopathic medicine called *Tuberculinum*, which is a preparation made from the infected lung tissue of a tuberculosis patient. It can be used to remove the chronic predisposition toward respiratory illnesses in individuals who have inherited the tubercular miasmatic influence. I have successfully used it many times in my own practice. The fact that it does work lends weight to the argument that this is not an irreversible genetic phenomenon, but rather an energetic one that can be mitigated if not completely removed.

Example 4

A woman who was viciously bitten by a dog and subsequently received rabies vaccine injections, later conceives a child who does not have rabies but who, nevertheless, displays many of the symptoms associated with "hydrophobia." The child acts fearful, is terrified of water, and can alternately act in an aggressive manner.

Here is another example of a miasmatic energetic influence. In a similar vein to the preceding tubercular miasm case, this case is an example of the rabies or hydrophobic miasm. Even though this woman did not actually contract rabies, her child exhibits symptoms that are commonly seen in those who are infected by rabies. Both the dog bite and the rabies vaccine are capable of inducing an energetic state that resembles rabies. It is possible for persons in the grip of this energetic state to transfer its influence to their offspring through birth.

As with *Tuberculinum* and tuberculosis, there is a homeopathic medicine called *Lyssinum*, which is made from the saliva of a rabid dog. When properly prescribed, it can remove symptoms that stem from such hydrophobic influences as animal bites or rabies vaccination. In this case, it would be a reasonable course of treatment for both mother and child.

Example 5

A man with a hot temper and a distinct craving for spicy foods brings a child into the world who, at an early age, displays a strikingly similar tendency to become angry at the slightest provocation and who, given his age, has an unusual taste for spicy foods.

I give this example simply to illustrate the idea that symptoms, quirks, and dysfunctional characteristics that cannot be attributed to genetics are capable of being transmitted to offspring. Even though we can discern no apparent originating cause for this man's anger issues, we still know that it is not a genetic trait. Rather, it is an energetic dysfunction of his vital force and, as such, is capable of being transmitted to his children.

The same applies to the spicy food craving. Although we would not necessarily call it a symptom, it can be a useful clue for constitutional prescribing. If a child had an uncontrollable desire for sweets, that would be viewed by a homeopath as a symptom that can lead in the long run to poor health. Proper treatment is capable of moderating cravings of this sort.

This also illustrates the very important point that some behaviors, such as the temper of this man's child, are not learned and not attributable to bad parenting. In other words, there is no one to blame. It is what it is, an unfortunate fate in life. Fortunately, energetic disturbances of this nature are capable of being remedied with proper homeopathic treatment. In this case, father and son are likely to benefit from the same constitutional remedy.

Epigenetics and bioenergetics

The scientific world is all abuzz these days over the exciting new field of epigenetics. The discovery of epigenetic markers have led scientists to conclude that traits previously thought not possible to transmit from one generation to the next are, in fact, capable of being inherited via a mechanism involving chemical modifiers that turn genes on and off. If true, such a discovery would turn everything conventional science knows about inheritance on its head. A recent article about epigenetic research at Mount Sinai Hospital in New York makes this field of inquiry sound very promising indeed:

> *Genetic changes stemming from the trauma suffered by Holocaust survivors are capable of being passed on to their children, the clearest sign yet that one person's life experience can affect subsequent generations. ... To our knowledge, this provides the first demonstration of transmission of pre-conception stress effects resulting in epigenetic changes in both the exposed parents and their offspring in humans...*[52]

If mainstream medicine had been paying any attention, it would have known that homeopathic physicians have been aware of this type of inheritance for more than two hundred years. Not only are homeopaths aware of this phenomenon, they have studied it in great detail from both theoretical and practical perspectives. They understand that all sorts of influences inimical to health can be transmitted—not via genetic or epigenetic mechanisms—but through *bioenergetic* means.

The bioenergetic imprints of emotional traumas, acute and chronic diseases, suppressive drug treatments, vaccinations, and much more can leave their mark on the individuals that they afflict. Those same factors can also leave their mark on offspring and even subsequent generations, creating predispositions toward illness that may or may not become manifest depending on various factors that encourage or discourage the expression of disease.

This remarkable body of homeopathic knowledge has been studiously ignored by mainstream medicine for a variety of grossly prejudicial reasons. The fault clearly lies with medicine's philosophical orientation. Medicine, in essence, is not willing to consider, examine, or study any phenomenon that is not supported by concrete physical evidence. This is why neuroscience focuses so much attention on the physical brain while ignoring the unexplored powers of the human psyche. As far as science is concerned, the psyche might as well not exist if it cannot be felt, smelt, seen, or heard.

In similar fashion, it was not permissible to entertain the possibility of non-genetic inheritance until epigenetics made the concept palatable to science's materialist sensibilities. The topic is no longer taboo in academic circles now that scientists have something concrete to point to. However, this new freedom to discuss non-traditional genetic inheritance is still hampered by the fact that it can only be conceptualized in concrete terms—epigenetic markers—once again causing medical science to miss the mark entirely.

Medicine's materialist bias causes it to routinely mistake association for causation. Contrary to what scientists now believe, epigenetic changes that modify gene expression are not the causes of inheritance. They are the result. *They are an outcome of bioenergetic inheritance.* Energetic factors beyond the understanding of conventional science cause changes in gene expression. This illustrates the profound and fundamental difference between conventional medicine and most forms of holism. While the one sees all things as a function of material forces, the other knows that all things are energetically connected.

Epigenetic manipulation of gene expression is a reductionist biotech fantasy that promises pots of gold at the end of the corporate rainbow. The danger of this type of wishful medical thinking is that it encourages risky interventions that don't always turn out as promised. Epigenetics is an opportunity waiting to be exploited by the biotech and nanotech industries, industries that have left a trail of environmental and human destruction. Although I am not arguing that biotech is all bad, its very existence is predicated upon financial gain, not human health.

The real reason why epigenetics has created such scientific fervor is because it represents yet another way that science gets to co-opt the psyche. Epigenetics gives medicine reason to claim ownership of consciousness on its own terms. It creates the illusion, as with brain science, that mind can be reduced, studied, and manipulated in material terms and by material means. It is just another foolish attempt by material science to co-opt the impenetrable mysteries of the human mind. When all is said and done, I suspect that the field of epigenetics will yield very little in terms of practical applications to human health. It will turn out to be a reductionist dead end.

The potential value of epigenetics is made moot by the fact that homeopathy has successfully employed the concept of energetic inheritance in the treatment of patients for two centuries. It is a new concept only to the conventional world of science.

A mother whose young child suffered from sleeplessness once consulted me. The child cried incessantly at night. I tried a few remedies that did little to help. During one of our meetings, the mother described a traumatic event that had occurred several years prior to the birth of her child. She had awoken one night to find an intruder at the foot of her bed. Thankfully, the intruder fled after she screamed. Of interest to me was the fact that she had left her body during this shocking event. She recalled the entire episode from the perspective of a person hovering above the bed, looking down upon the scene at herself and the intruder. She could still see the event vividly in her head, as if she were watching a movie.

This turned out to be the critical bit of information that I needed. I prescribed a remedy known to fit the effects of traumatic events of a shocking or frightening nature. It can also be used to help people whose health problems can be traced to out-of-body experiences. A couple doses of the remedy immediately settled the child down. The crying ceased and everyone in the house was able to sleep peacefully. (Remedy choice?[53])

Here we have an example of a mental-emotional-sleep problem that clearly was not genetically inherited. Neither was it epigenetically induced; it was energetically induced. There is a reason why we use the word "shock" when referring to such experiences. While it may be true that the shocking incident could possibly have altered the epigenetic expression of the mother, *the trauma itself and the consequences that were passed on to the child were energetic in nature.*

If it were even possible to design a drug to chemically flip the epigenetic switches on genes supposedly involved in the transference of trauma, the problem would not likely be solved (never mind the side effects that would result). The most a chemical intervention can accomplish when dealing with an energetic phenomenon is to keep a temporary lid on the situation. While symptoms may be suppressed, the underlying energetic disturbance in the vital force remains. Health problems created by energetic imbalances can only be resolved by energetic interventions.

Returning now to the topic of how we get sick, we can see that there are a multitude of factors that contribute to illness. Our predispositions toward certain types of illnesses are determined by a complex combination of our *genetic* makeup, our *energetic* inheritance, and the many *environmental* factors that influence our lives. While some disease factors are genetically hardwired, most are not. When homeopaths refer to miasms and miasmatic influences, they are talking about those factors that are energetically acquired or inherited. Since all individuals inherit energetic influences that have been passed down through the generations, and since such influences are amenable to homeopathic intervention, a clear understanding of the topic is of great significance to all who seek healing for what ails them.

A word about disease causation

While I covered this topic at length in my previous books, it bears repeating because of its importance. Conventional medicine has sown a great deal of confusion over the causes of disease. The same is also true of many holistic theories of disease. In truth, it is almost impossible to pin down single causes for particular illnesses. As discussed above, illness is a complex interplay of many factors. The notion that science can isolate individual causes of disease is a delusion made possible by its myopic worldview. More importantly, solutions for illnesses that come from such a narrow perspective almost always fall short of the mark, and frequently result in unforeseen consequences.

When mainstream medicine leads us to believe that cholesterol-clogged arteries cause heart attacks, it reduces a multifactorial problem to one oversimplified factor. Likewise, when it blames an infection on a particular virus or bacterium, it leaves out all other factors that make people susceptible to microbial colonization. We know that reaming out a clogged artery does not solve heart disease. We also know that repeatedly killing a bacterium that supposedly caused an infection tends to render one more susceptible to further infections, and those infections are less likely to respond to additional antibiotics the more they are used.

If this is true, then something must be wrong with our understanding of disease causation. Many conventional theories of disease causation are reductionist explanations that confuse causation with association. While it is true that constricted airways are associated with asthma, they are not the cause of asthma. While it is true that vascular congestion is associated with certain types of migraines, it is not the cause of such migraines. While drugs aimed at these supposed causes may bring temporary relief, they will not prevent future episodes of asthma or migraines. The true causes of these conditions run deep and are far more complex than medical science acknowledges.

Most disease causes proposed by conventional medical science are not true causes. More often, they are just associated phenomena. Sometimes they are factors that act as disease triggers, but not true causes. Peanut consumption may trigger an allergic response but peanuts are not the cause of that person's allergy. The true cause of such problems has more to do with the individual person's constitutional circumstances than with peanuts. This is not to ignore the reality that some people's health issues can be compounded by the consumption of peanuts. The point is that many who consume peanuts enjoy good health while others do not. The true source of the problem, therefore, is a function of a complex combination of bioenergetic, constitutional, and environmental factors.

It is easy to be dazzled by the authoritative voice of medical science when it proposes definitive explanations of disease causation in highly complex language. Do not be fooled by such scientific lingo. It is best to view all reductionist theories of disease causation with a critical eye. Any disease theory that fails to take into account the whole person, by definition, focuses on certain factors while ignoring many others. Treatments based on such theories must yield only partial or temporary results.

Orthodox medicine's bias predisposes it to favor the idea of single isolated material causes for most illnesses. Thus, brain neurotransmitters are responsible for depression, germs cause infections, genes are suspected to be the reason for many illnesses that have yet to be explained and, now, epigenetic factors are becoming a favored explanation for mental illness.

Holism, in essence, is the opposite of reductionism. While reductionism looks for single isolated material causes and solutions, holism always takes into account the broadest possible perspective. Homeopathy is perhaps the most all-encompassing holistic approach to illness ever devised. Homeopathy understands the difference between a simple trigger that provokes an episode of illness and the multitude of contributing factors that can lead to a predisposition to that illness.

Homeopathy also understands that true causation is something that can never be fully known. On the spectrum of causation, orthodox medicine always chooses proximate causation, which is the one factor that is closest in time and space to the most recent flare-up of an illness. On the opposite end of the spectrum is ultimate or final causation. While it may not be possible to definitively determine ultimate causation, it remains true that the closer one comes to addressing the deepest underlying causes of disease, the better the therapeutic outcome will be.

For example, when an adult receives a diagnosis of rheumatoid arthritis (RA), the physician knows that the only conventional option is to address the presumed underlying physical cause. A variety of powerful drugs can be prescribed to combat the autoimmune inflammatory response that is believed to be the cause of this illness. No one expects the illness to be cured. Everyone knows that RA is a lifelong condition that will need to be managed with ongoing drug therapy.

The homeopath, on the other hand, understands that inflammation is not the cause of RA. Depending upon how you look at it, inflammation is either a process associated with RA, a way to describe RA, or the end result of RA. But inflammation is not the cause of RA.

A thorough and comprehensive physical, mental, emotional, environmental, and historical investigation often reveals the deeper causes of conditions like RA. It's not hard to do; it simply requires that one connect the dots. For example, it is possible to trace a case of RA to an episode of the flu during which the person experienced joint pains, among other symptoms. That person admits to never having fully shaken the flu until one day, a few months later, the joint pains intensify, leading to a diagnosis of rheumatoid arthritis. As previously described, this case of RA could be attributed to having *never been well since the flu*.

Another person notes that the sudden death of his brother caused him tremendous grief. He acknowledges that he has internalized that grief and is not inclined to talk about it. In fact, he also notes that this is typical of his *modus operandi*. He also has not dealt with the internal grief that came from the death of his mother five years earlier. Six months after his brother's passing he began to experience joint pains, which ultimately led to a diagnosis of RA. Here, it is reasonable to conclude that the deeper cause of RA is unresolved grief.

Now, imagine what happens when drug therapy designed to combat inflammation is the main approach to this case of RA. Isn't it reasonable to conclude that while it may provide temporary symptomatic relief, the underlying grief will continue to smolder, thus causing the RA to persist? Even worse, it may contribute to the development of deeper manifestations of illness. To reduce RA to a simple matter of inflammation is a naïve assumption that can lead to a great deal of harm.

I could go on with many more examples of how or why people develop rheumatoid arthritis. Suffice it to say, the potential causes are complex, varied, and oftentimes multifactorial. The bottom line is that just about anything can cause anything. There are no hard fast rules. Every situation is unique. No one person's life circumstances are like any other person's life circumstances. The genetic heritage, energetic inheritance, psychological makeup, and life experiences of each individual constitute the breeding ground upon which illness either takes root or does not take root.

Suppression and iatrogenesis

There is perhaps no greater contributing factor to the development of chronic disease than allopathic medicine itself. Iatrogenesis, or medically induced disease, is a well-known phenomenon. To its credit, conventional medicine acknowledges the role of iatrogenesis when it admits, for example, to the side effects of drugs, botched surgeries, hospital acquired infections, allergic reactions, and adverse events related to diagnostic procedures. However, from a homeopathic perspective this represents only a small fraction of the problem.

The greatest source of chronic disease is allopathic treatment itself. By this, I do not mean treatment gone awry. I am referring to successful treatment, treatment that has achieved its intended goal. Since medicine's reductionist philosophy allows it to see only one small piece of the larger holistic puzzle at a time, it remains insulated from the larger implications of its treatment strategies. Orthodox medicine has perfected the art of targeted short-term treatment. It must content itself with temporary relief from localized symptoms because that is the best that it has to offer. The problem is that suppressive methods inevitably lead to chronic illness. Conventional medicine lacks the philosophical perspective and requisite therapeutic tools to handle illness in ways that do not increase the probability of further harm.

Doctors and patients alike tend to assume that they know what the term *suppression* means. Sadly, this is just not true. Since suppression is the driving force behind the rising incidence of chronic disease around the globe, I believe that homeopathic practitioners have an obligation to increase awareness of this phenomenon in the clearest terms possible.

When asked, the average person is likely to describe suppression in immunologic terms. In other words, it is believed to be a type of weakening of the immune system, which can result in greater susceptibility to microbial invasion. While this is partially true, it fails to take into account the larger role of suppression. Suppression needs to be understood in its much broader context.

No symptom, no matter how superficial or odd, is random. All homeopaths begin with this basic understanding—each symptom has a purpose within the greater whole of the human organism. Although that purpose may not always be discernable, all symptoms must be seen in the larger context as expressions of imbalance of the underlying vital life energy that animates each human being.

Symptoms can manifest on any or all levels: physical, emotional, mental, and spiritual. When the life force is unhappy, it generates symptoms that reflect its degree of distress. Diarrhea, for example, is a more serious sign of distress than, say, a runny nose. A tendency to jealous rage is a more serious symptom than a flare-up of hemorrhoids. It is possible for symptoms to jump from one level to another. The energetic focus of a condition can shift, for example, from migraines to anxiety and back to migraines again. The manner in which symptoms are expressed depends upon the overall health of the vital force. Herein lies the limitation of conventional medical understanding, which fails to take seriously the unity of body and mind and the reality of the life force.

A comparatively healthy life force will tend to generate more superficial, less threatening symptoms, such as sneezing, temporary sadness, or a patch of itchy skin. A more compromised life force will often generate more serious acute symptoms, such as sudden facial paralysis or intense abdominal pain, or chronic symptoms, such as loss of interest in life or arthritic hip pain.

When we understand the above, it becomes clear why most normal healthy babies tend to get diaper rashes, runny noses, and fevers. In contrast, less healthy adults tend to complain of symptoms such as headaches, stiff joints, and bouts of sleeplessness. Adults with more compromised states of health tend to develop high blood pressure, chronic fatigue, and mood disorders like depression or anxiety. The skyrocketing incidence of chronic illness in Western societies is disquieting, and appears to be affecting not just adults but younger people, too.

So what accounts for the difference between healthy adults and chronically ill adults, or healthy and not so healthy kids for that matter? This trend, in my opinion, is a direct consequence of the frequency with which we resort to pharmacological and surgical solutions. The outcomes, in terms of who remains healthy and whose health deteriorates over time, are not at all random. Long-term health is almost a direct function of the way in which symptoms and illnesses are managed. Suppressive treatments tend to result in unfavorable long-term outcomes. When we consider that almost all conventional approaches to illness are fundamentally suppressive, the implications for our collective health are alarming.

The life force generates symptoms as a coping mechanism. They represent the life force's best efforts to heal itself. The vast majority of the time, this self-healing mechanism works just fine without outside intervention—most conditions resolve on their own after their purposes have been served. Medical culture has conditioned us, however, to have little tolerance for the discomfort of symptoms. We reach for pharmaceutical solutions the moment symptoms appear. If we only understood the true nature of symptoms and their purpose, we might be inclined to make healthier choices regarding their treatment.

Conventional drugs have one purpose only, and that is to extinguish symptoms. Herein lies the problem. The life force produces symptoms in order to survive. Drugs are used to prevent those very same symptoms. Drugs are not designed to heal or to assist the life force. When drugs suppress symptoms, they work at cross-purposes with the life force. When the life force is deprived of one particular avenue of expression, it chooses the next best way to vent its distress. The next best avenue of expression often takes the form of symptoms that are less desirable and more threatening than the original symptoms.

Suppression drives illness deeper into the system, causing it to morph into more serious problems. The life force manifests its distress in the most favorable way possible, given the parameters of each situation. A strong life force will focus its energy toward the periphery, thus generating relatively superficial symptoms such as a simple skin eruption or a runny nose. As the life force weakens and becomes compromised, illness manifests on deeper levels.

It should come as no surprise, then, when a person develops depression for the first time after having successfully controlled his asthma with steroid-based inhalers. Likewise, it is no coincidence when a young child develops an ear infection after her diaper rash has been suppressed with zinc oxide cream. In each case, the life force must choose a second, less desirable way to express the energetic imbalance that led to symptoms in the first place.

As a general rule, there is a hierarchical relationship in terms of the way illness manifests in the human organism. It proceeds from less compromising to more compromising symptomatology. It also proceeds roughly in this direction: from physical > to emotional > to mental > to spiritual. When drug therapy successfully targets a certain set of physical symptoms, thus preventing their expression, the life force often redirects the disturbance to another, less desirable physical location. When physical symptoms are repeatedly suppressed, there is a tendency for the disturbance to eventually "metastasize" to another, deeper level. When forced away from the physical level, the energetic disturbance often resurfaces on the mental or emotional levels. Since conventional medicine does not acknowledge this phenomenon, it is spared from taking responsibility for the role it plays in generating mental, emotional, and spiritual illness.

Most drugs are designed to suppress the most immediate symptoms without regard for their impact on the greater whole or their longer-term consequences. A painkiller may dull a headache but it is not likely to promote healing. Tylenol may lower a fever but it is not necessarily in the best interest of overall health. Cortisone can make eczema disappear but this is done at the risk of one's long-term health. While truly threatening symptoms may necessitate temporary suppressive measures, most illnesses do not fall into this category. Conventional medicine makes no distinction and, by default, opts for a suppressive approach in almost all cases, regardless of the level of threat.

The overall impact of iatrogenic side effects and adverse events in medicine pales in comparison to the degree to which suppression encourages the development of chronic disease. This is the real untold story of medicine's propensity for undermining long-term health.

Genuine healing works in a direction opposite to suppression. Any truly effective healing method is always cognizant of the greater whole and longer-term trends in health status. Homeopathy respects the wisdom of the body and seeks to work with symptoms of illness rather than against them, thereby contributing to positive long-term outcomes.

Beware of the worst iatrogenic offenders

Although all drugs suppress symptoms, a great deal of iatrogenic harm can be traced to three particular classes of drugs. Antimicrobials, steroids, and vaccines are responsible for the rise in chronic disease more so than other drugs, largely because of their widespread and frequent use.

Antimicrobials

Needless to say, this class of drugs is prescribed far too frequently. Antimicrobials can disrupt the balance of the body's internal microenvironment. In the process of killing so-called "bad bugs," the human body's normal flora is also impacted. Most people are regularly exposed to dietary doses of antibiotics by virtue of their heavy use in animal husbandry. While probiotics can be helpful, they don't necessarily restore the body to its prior state of microbial balance.

Another well-documented issue is the way in which antibiotics encourage natural selection of germs that are resistant to treatment, thus speeding up the evolutionary development of bacteria that are more dangerous and harder to eradicate. Medical authorities acknowledge the issue of bacterial resistance but fail to make use of alternatives like homeopathy. The same concept applies to antifungals and antivirals. If you think bacterial "superbugs" are a problem, just wait until the over-prescription of antivirals are blamed for the appearance of super viruses. While antibiotics are necessary and valuable tools in every doctor's kit, they should be used only when necessary.

Perhaps the most common example of the hazards of overuse can be seen in children with chronic ear infections. These poor kids just seem to get sicker with each new round of antibiotics taken. The average kid taking antibiotics for his or her fifth, sixth, or seventh ear infection tends to look pale, sickly, and frail. The child's appetite, mood, and vitality are often adversely affected. While this is partially due to the ear infections, it is also a function of the antibiotics themselves. Antibiotics can be effective in the short run, but they encourage the recurrence of infections and weaken the immune system in the long run. More important, the vicious cycle of antibiotic overuse contributes to the emergence of additional, more problematic health issues. Antimicrobials are a significant factor in the development of chronic physical, mental, and emotional illness.

Fortunately, there is a reliable alternative to antibiotics. For many years, I have successfully used homeopathy to treat all types of viral and bacterial infections, including colds, flus, ear infections, conjunctivitis, sinusitis, tonsillitis, laryngitis, bronchitis, pneumonia, dental abscesses, cellulitis, urinary tract infections, and more. While it is true that homeopathic treatment can boost immunity, this is an oversimplification. Homeopathy works not by killing germs, but by rousing the vital force to resist germs that take advantage of weaknesses created by a variety of factors.

It is reasonable to assume that 50% of all antibiotic prescriptions could be avoided if physicians were properly trained in acute care homeopathy. I believe that percentage would rise to 75% or higher if most people received constitutional homeopathic care. Then, antibiotic treatment could be reserved as a last resort, to be used only when necessary. Homeopathy reduces the need for antibiotics, restores health to those harmed by antibiotic overuse, and prevents the development of drug-resistant germs, thereby preserving the effectiveness of antibiotics for when they are truly needed.

Corticosteroids

This is a class of steroid hormone-based drugs that includes over-the-counter topical cortisone cream, hydrocortisone, and prednisone. The medical establishment makes no bones about what these drugs are; they are openly referred to as immunosuppressant drugs. Their use is on the rise for one very good reason; they appear to work as if by magic. They are extremely powerful drugs that can quickly obliterate most symptoms that they target. Rub a little cortisone on a rash and, poof, it's gone! Inject some cortisone into that achy joint and, voila, it's like new! Doctors and patients love steroids because they suppress symptoms so effectively.

But therein lies the danger. When a drug like cortisone snuffs out symptoms as ruthlessly as it does, it would be naïve not to expect a backlash from the life force. That backlash may come quickly or can occur at a later date. When the backlash is delayed, neither patient nor doctor is inclined to trace it back to the steroids. Corticosteroids are dangerous precisely because they work so well.

For example, when arthritic pain located in the right shoulder disappears after a cortisone injection but then returns six months later, the patient should consider him or herself lucky. In such a case, the life force had enough resilience to keep the problem confined to the original site. If, on the other hand, the right shoulder remains well but a similar pain shows up in the left shoulder three months later, that is not a good sign. In such a case, although the life force manages to keep the affliction on the physical level, it has redirected it to a new location. While a conventional doctor might interpret this as an unavoidable spread of the arthritis that the cortisone was unable to contain, a homeopath sees this as a direct consequence of inappropriate suppressive treatment. A backlash was likely; it was just a matter of when and where it would manifest.

Now, let's say that the right shoulder pain disappears after a cortisone shot but the patient then develops pneumonia three weeks later. The pneumonia resolves with antibiotics, but difficulty with breathing persists. A new diagnosis of asthma is made and the patient is instructed to take two new medications to help keep the problem under control. In this case, the life force has been weakened to such an extent that it must retreat and draw a new line of defense in the lungs where it manifests its distress as asthma.

Another patient receives the same cortisone injection for right shoulder pain. Two months later, she experiences a significant change in mood. After consulting her physician, she receives a new diagnosis of depression and is prescribed an antidepressant. Here we see a shift of the disturbance from the physical to the mental-emotional level.

There is no limit to the potential responses of the vital force to such a powerful and suppressive treatment as cortisone. Corticosteroids are known for a wide range of serious side effects. But it is misleading to call them side effects. They cannot be thought of as routine unwanted symptoms that one must endure in order to experience the so-called beneficial effects. They are more accurately characterized as the indirect but expected compensatory response to the suppression of target symptoms.

In my medical opinion, corticosteroids are a dangerous class of drugs responsible for a great deal of serious and sometimes life-threatening illness. On the one hand, they have become drugs of last resort, to be prescribed when doctors have nothing left to offer. On the other hand, steroid creams are now available over-the-counter, thus giving the public the false impression that they are benign. The fact that they come in topical form in no way mitigates their potential for harm. Again, in my opinion, to play with these drugs is to play with fire. I make a point of cautioning all my patients that corticosteroids are drugs of absolute last resort.

Although the successful suppression of symptoms is far more common with corticosteroids, the same basic concept applies to all drugs. Most drugs are suppressive by their very nature. They are purposely designed to prevent symptoms from manifesting. The more successfully a drug accomplishes that goal, the greater is its potential for creating unwanted consequences. Any drug that can suppress symptoms has the potential to cause a decline in overall health.

Homeopathy is a viable alternative for many of the problems that are now routinely treated with corticosteroids. While some of these conditions, such as asthma and colitis, may require significant time commitments in order to achieve homeopathic success, this is preferable to the risks of immunosuppressive treatment. Homeopathy is a far safer alternative that promotes overall long-term well-being.

Vaccines

Although a great deal more can be written about vaccination, I will make my comments brief. Vaccines are not a source of suppression as much as they represent a direct assault upon the immune system. In my medical opinion, they are the greatest of all causes of iatrogenic autoimmune disease. In spite of this reality, governments of many developed countries in cahoots with industry mandate that vaccines be administered to all children. Disturbingly, there are rumblings indicating that the mandate will eventually be extended to include adults, too.

There is an abundance of evidence that points to the fact that vaccines can trigger eczema, allergies, asthma, seizures, neurologic disorders, encephalopathy, learning disabilities, attention and hyperactivity problems, psychiatric disorders and, yes, even autism. The rising incidence of these chronic diseases in American children is terrifying.

The scientific community is being deliberately obtuse when it denies the link between vaccines and these illnesses. The truth is that current law protects vaccine manufacturers from all liability. In 1986, the U.S. government created a vaccine injury compensation fund—National Vaccine Injury Compensation Program (NVICP)—specifically to appease vaccine manufacturers who were reluctant to market their products. The very act of compensating individuals for vaccine injuries is an admission of the harm that vaccinations can cause. The Vaccine Adverse Event Reporting System (VAERS) keeps an official record of all known adverse events. This information is available online for consumers to view. Even medical authorities admit that there are many more such events that never get reported.

It is in the interests of government and the scientific community to prevent the truth regarding vaccines from reaching the mainstream. The root cause of this scandal is the arrogance of scientific authority and its general contempt for patients whose pleas for common sense have gone unheeded. The audacity of the medical community to argue that the evidence provided by parents who witness adverse vaccine events in their children is just "anecdotal" information, and not real evidence, is beyond reprehensible.

The number of required vaccines has steadily risen over the course of time and shows no sign of slowing down. I believe that we will someday look back at this era of immunologic experimentation via compulsory vaccination as the greatest medical scandal of all time. The devastation wrought will be beyond compare.

I should emphasize that these are my personal beliefs regarding vaccines based upon my medical training and my experiences as a physician. Technically, my position has nothing to do with homeopathy and does not necessarily represent the beliefs of other homeopathic practitioners. With that said, homeopathy has a very long track record of successful treatment of vaccine-induced health problems. In homeopathy, vaccine-related illness is referred to as *vaccinosis*. Homeopaths have been aware of and have treated vaccinosis for over a hundred years.

Furthermore, the main purpose of vaccines is to *prevent* diseases that have little to no effective conventional treatment. The medical establishment is not interested in the fact that homeopathy has a long history of having successfully treated those very same illnesses *after they have been contracted*. Medical and hospital records from the 1800s provide irrefutable evidence of this success. The amazing thing is that the same homeopathic treatment options are still available today to those who contract any one of these diseases. The fear factor regarding epidemic disease diminishes significantly when one has homeopathic treatment to assist in recovery.

When we consider the suppressive influence of drugs and the spectrum of illness caused by vaccines, the concept of iatrogenesis extends far beyond its original conventional definition. Drugs work by short-circuiting, preventing, and suppressing the efforts of the life force to heal itself. Although sometimes necessary in emergent situations, suppression as a general strategic approach to illness inevitably leads to declining health and chronic illness.

Susceptibility to disease

The greatest determinant of personal health, *individual susceptibility*, is a topic that is sorely neglected by the medical establishment. Medicine focuses its attention on external factors while ignoring the role of the "host." For example, not everyone exposed to the flu bug comes down with the flu. Some are susceptible while others are not. It's not the germ that causes the illness as much as the susceptibility of the life force to the influence of the germ. Medicine obsesses about germs but shows little interest in learning why germ-resistant individuals have the capacity to resist germs.

Illness is not something that invades from the outside. It develops from the inside. It's not the various stressors that cause us to become sick. It has more to do with the way that we handle those stressors, which, in turn, is a function of the health status of the life force. A weakened life force is more susceptible to the influences of life's stresses. A healthy person can go snow skiing in cold windy weather without consequence. Another person develops bronchitis from the same activity. A strong and healthy life force can withstand the verbal assault of an abusive person. A weaker life force may express its response to such abuse by generating migraines or by plunging the person into depression.

All illness can ultimately be attributed to a disturbance in the life force. In this sense, illness begins on the inside and then manifests on the periphery as discernable symptomatology. The externally observable symptoms are but a reflection of the interior status of some type of bioenergetic imbalance. It is an illusion to think that an illness can be located in a specific part or parts simply because that is where the symptoms are found. All symptoms point to an underlying issue involving the whole person. Homeopathic luminary, Herbert Roberts, MD, expressed this concept here, in his own words, almost a hundred years ago:

> ...we must acknowledge that disturbance of any part is the manifestation of an inner disturbance ... that it is an expression of the whole disturbance manifesting itself perhaps locally or in seemingly unrelated parts; it is an expression of the disturbed vital energy, and is a manifestation of the man as a unit, and not of the separate parts of his body. That brings us to the point of looking upon disease as a dynamic expression of the disturbance of the harmony and rhythm of the vital energy.[54]

When consulted by a person with an allergy, I often explain that the allergen is not the cause of the problem. Granted, allergens can trigger dysfunctional symptomatic responses in sensitive individuals, but the true source of the problem lies in the reaction of the life force to the allergen. The goal of treatment is not so much to avoid the allergen as it is to restore the strength of the vital force to the point where the person is no longer susceptible to the allergen. The same concept applies to food allergies, environmental allergies, and even exaggerated reactions to insect stings. True healing involves restoring balance to an out-of-balance life force. It is not possible to accomplish this via allergy shots, which are designed to desensitize the patient to allergens. This would constitute an unnatural form of tinkering with the immune system.

Remember that a person gets sick in the most advantageous way available to the life force, in a way that creates the least suffering. All of the aforementioned factors—genetic makeup, bioenergetically inherited influences, allopathic suppression, immunologic tinkering, and life's circumstances—together, determine the degree to which each unique individual is susceptible to illness. A healthy life force will express illness in a more superficial and less threatening manner. The more compromised the life force, the deeper the illness is likely to manifest.

The range of susceptibility of a healthy child is skewed toward conditions like rashes, colds, coughs, and ear infections. If the child's health declines, the range of susceptibility can shift in the direction of deeper, more problematic health issues such as insomnia, asthma, mood disorders, and behavioral problems. The child is no longer able to generate a simple run-of-the-mill cold that lasts a few days and resolves on its own. Instead, the child develops a thick yellow nasal discharge that does not clear up on its own. A pediatrician diagnoses sinusitis and prescribes an antibiotic, thereby perpetuating the vicious cycle of suppression.

People's hereditary influences and life circumstances are always unique. These factors form the soil, the terrain upon which physical, mental, and emotional health problems develop. Given the infinite number of factors that can impinge upon the life force, it's not surprising that health status and susceptibility to different forms of illness will vary tremendously from person to person.

Joe's grandfather survived combat in the World War before giving birth to Joe's father. Joe's father had high blood pressure and died of a heart attack. Joe's mother was always sick as a child, and as an adult was prone to pneumonia. Joe had his tonsils removed as a child, sustained a concussion during football practice in middle school, was given prednisone for an allergic reaction to a bee sting in high school, and experienced a significant blow to his self-esteem when he was not accepted into the college that he always dreamed of attending.

Now compare Joe to Katie whose grandparents almost died on the ship that brought them to America but allowed them to escape famine in their home country as teenagers. Katie's mother was sexually abused by an uncle, and her father ran off with a mistress, leaving the family financially destitute. Katie was sick a lot as a child, missed a lot of school, and had to repeat ninth grade. She developed chronic neck pain after a car accident in tenth grade, had her appendix surgically removed in eleventh grade, and shortly thereafter turned to alcohol as a means of coping with her problems.

It would be naïve to think that Joe and Katie's unique life circumstances would not impact the trajectory of their health over the course of their lifetimes. It's not hard to see how generationally inherited influences, along with various stressors and adverse circumstances over the course of one's lifetime, can impose layers of dysfunction upon the vital force. All of these factors combined determine the degree of the life force's susceptibility to various illnesses. It also illustrates the futility of cookie-cutter medicine, which tries to impose its one-size-fits-all treatments on people who have widely diverse life circumstances and hereditary backgrounds. The entire premise of homeopathy is predicated on understanding the interplay of those diverse factors and the impact they have on health and illness.

Expression of disease

Orthodox medicine places tremendous emphasis on diagnostic labeling. As I have argued elsewhere, the real reason behind this preoccupation with the diagnostic name game has to do with the relative lack of truly effective treatments at medicine's disposal. Since its treatment options are limited, medicine busies itself instead with diagnostic technicalities. Nowadays, most breakthroughs in medicine have to do with new technologies or lab tests, which allow doctors to detect clues that enable them to confirm diagnoses.

The media and general public are smitten by such diagnostic advances. But when was the last time you heard about a genuine breakthrough involving a truly effective treatment for some illness? Medicine's inability to think outside the box leaves it holding the same old therapeutic bag of tricks. As a result, medicine's version of "new" translates into marketing gimmicks like gel caps and extended-release dosing, and off-label uses for well-known drugs.

When you think about it, diagnostic labeling is really just a way of generalizing about patients and standardizing their treatments. Although there are legitimate purposes for diagnostic labeling, one of its unstated functions is to enable the implementation of cookie-cutter medicine. This treatment strategy is based on the ill-founded assumption that all people who fall into a given disease category should respond to the same therapeutic protocol.

This constitutes one of the more problematic flaws of modern medicine. It believes that uniformity and homogeneity are signs of scientific integrity. A successful diagnosis is one that conforms to the stereotypical ideal. It is considered scientifically sound because it satisfies the reproducibility and broad applicability criteria of science. The true unspoken purpose of diagnostic uniformity, however, is to serve the profit motive; it enables drugs to be marketed to large populations.

Reproducibility in medicine is the belief that a desirable treatment is one that can be applied to many individuals who fit the same diagnostic criteria. Treatments that can be administered to large populations garner greater interest than individualized approaches. This is not a requirement for good science as much as it is a bias of corporate medical science. Reproducibility is not an inherent feature of scientific method. It is a value imposed upon science by contemporary scientists. The net effect of this type of unscientific thinking is to stifle innovation.

Modern science is so blinded by this bias that it makes it incapable of comprehending homeopathy's individualized approach to treatment. Homeopaths understand that the ways in which illnesses manifest are virtually limitless. No one person's migraines are exactly like any other's. It makes little sense to homeopaths to lump people into artificially homogenized categories for the purposes of therapeutic convenience.

Diagnostic labels are distortions of holistic reality. They serve the purposes of the medical establishment more than the needs of patients. The goal of a homeopathic interview is to ascertain the reality of the patient's condition in its truest form, to understand the illness through the eyes of the patient without passing judgment and without reducing the patient's complaints to a prefabricated diagnostic category. When we take illness at face value, exactly as it is, it serves to validate the experiences of patients. It also increases the likelihood that they will receive the medical care that suits their actual needs. A successful prescription should not require that the physician see the patient as a stereotype. It demands that patients be understood on their own terms, inside and out.

In the same way that a multitude of factors create unique predispositions toward certain types of illness, so, too, the way in which we express those illnesses is highly unique and variable. Different people express the "same" illness in completely different ways. This is the crux, the entire point of homeopathy.

For example, let's take three different people of the same age, each of whom has just lost their mother to the same type of cancer. The first person weeps and wails uncontrollably and is virtually unable to function given the volatility of her emotions. Six months later, she continues to grieve, breaking down into sobbing fits at unpredictable moments. Her emotions continue to wreak havoc in her life. (Remedy choice?[55])

The second person takes the event very seriously, is devastated by the loss, and begins to question the nature of life and existence. She prays for guidance but gradually sinks into a deep depression. She questions how this could have happened and begins to lose her faith. She debates whether there really is a God and starts to experience fleeting suicidal thoughts. (Remedy choice?[56])

A third person appears to grieve initially but then gradually sinks into a depressed funk. He begins to sleep excessively, unable to drag himself out of bed in the morning. When awake, he sits around watching TV, disinterested in his usual activities and disinclined to socialize. Six months later, he admits to feeling a type of apathetic numbness. He complains of fatigue and lack of motivation. (Remedy choice?[57])

Here we have three completely different manifestations of the effects of grief and loss. There are many more that I could describe, but these three will serve for this example. All three represent unique expressions of the vital force in distress. All three are a function of cumulative factors that predispose each person to manifest his or her grief in different ways. There is no right way or wrong way. It serves no purpose to tell a stoic person to cry or a hysterical person to get a grip. They all represent involuntary responses to grief that have become stuck.

A healthy response is one that allows a person to pass through the various phases of grief without getting bogged down in any one phase for a prolonged period of time. Unfortunately, for a variety of predisposing reasons, many are not able to overcome the trauma of grief. Such persons could benefit greatly from homeopathic intervention.

The very same factors that predispose one to illness—genetic makeup, bioenergetic influences, allopathic suppression, and so on—also play a role in the manner in which illness is expressed. One such factor is encapsulated by the notion of "types." If you are an observant person, it should come as no surprise that people come in all types. There are distinct and discernable body types just as there are unique personality types. Homeopathy recognizes that different types of people tend to express illnesses in ways that are typical of their type.

This is where the concept of "constitutional" medicine comes from. A constitutional *Silica* type tends to be tall, thin, and emotionally reserved. Such persons tend to express digestive dysfunction in the form of constipation. Constitutional *Sulphur* types tend to be warm-blooded, disorganized, and have a preference for hot spicy foods. These types are likely to express digestive troubles in the form of diarrhea that acts up especially in the mornings. Not all persons fit such neatly defined constitutional types. Nevertheless, the concept of types illustrates the idea that who we are defines how we get sick.

Taking the idea of types a step further, all homeopaths know that disease patterns are reflective of patterns that already exist in nature. There is nothing new under the sun. Humanity and its ailments are inextricably woven into the fabric of nature. This is why homeopathy holds such promise for so many common and uncommon illnesses. It is aware of the fact that healing can be achieved by matching the symptom pattern of the suffering patient to the symptom pattern of some substance in nature.

People get sick in ways that mirror nature. Put another way, archetypal energies that inform patterns in nature also inform patterns of illness. It is not unusual to find substances from different kingdoms that mirror each other and that mirror our illnesses. For example, the remedy *Ignatia amara* is of the plant kingdom. *Natrum muriaticum* is a mineral remedy. The two can easily be confused and are commonly prescribed for problems that arise from the trauma of grief. In other words, human grief can reflect and induce symptom patterns produced by substances from both the plant and mineral kingdoms.

I do believe that the eminent biologist, Rupert Sheldrake, would do well to explore the theory and applications of homeopathy. He would find a striking resemblance between certain aspects of homeopathy and his theories regarding morphic fields and morphic resonance. In his own words:

> *My own hypothesis is that the formation of habits depend on a process called morphic resonance. Similar patterns of activity resonate across time and space with subsequent patterns. This hypothesis applies to all self-organizing systems, including atoms, molecules, crystals, cells, plants, animals and animal societies. All draw upon a collective memory and in turn contribute to it. ... Morphic fields are shaped by morphic resonance from all similar past systems, and thus contain a cumulative collective memory. Morphic resonance depends on similarity, and is not attenuated by distance in space or time. Morphic fields are local, within and around the systems they organize, but morphic resonance is non-local.*[58]

I'll leave it up to Professor Sheldrake and other scientists to wrangle over the mechanism by which such phenomena occur. Suffice it to say that it does occur and homeopathy is living proof that resonance is a guiding principle of the natural world. It is no coincidence that we get sick in patterns similar to the patterns produced by substances from animal, vegetable, and mineral kingdoms.

While we all get sick in our own unique ways, the process is not random. There are detectable and sometimes predictable patterns. Discerning such patterns is the expertise of the homeopathic practitioner. Conventional medicine generalizes by compartmentalizing illnesses based on broad commonalities that strip each individual case of its unique identifying characteristics. While it can be helpful for a homeopath to know the general nature of a patient's condition, effective prescribing requires much more detailed information.

Let's try another example. Each of the following patients has been diagnosed as having gastroenteritis. However, each has a uniquely different symptom pattern. The details in each case are what enable a homeopathic prescriber to choose a medicine based on the principle of similars.

The first patient has fever, chills, and both vomiting and diarrhea. Her vomiting is frequent and violent and the degree of fluid loss makes the possibility of dehydration a real concern. There is no complaint of pain. She is exhausted from the experience. She also has a peculiar combination of symptoms in that she feels icy cold and yet craves ice cold drinks. She also has a desire to suck on ice pops. (Remedy choice?[59])

A second person also has fever, chills, and vomiting. However, in this case the patient complains mostly about nausea and abdominal cramps. Even after emptying his stomach contents, he continues to retch in a spasmodic manner. He feels very chilly and acts quite irritable. It turns out that he indulged heavily in rich food, coffee, and alcohol the night before the illness began. (Remedy choice?[60])

A third patient has a fever and had one episode of vomiting, but her main complaint is diarrhea. The diarrhea tends to be worse early in the mornings, driving her out of bed and into the bathroom. She complains of feeling quite warm, so much so that she slept without any covers the night before. She complains of a burning pain in the stomach. (Remedy choice?[61])

Again, we see here how different people express the same illness differently. They are considered the same illness only from the artificially constructed perspective of conventional medical diagnostics. There is little that medicine has to offer in such cases other than supportive measures such as bed rest and hydration. Although these conditions are treatable from a homeopathic perspective, each represents a completely different illness that requires individual attention.

Taking into account body type, personality type, genetic history, bioenergetic inheritance, personal life events, family environment, socio-economic influences, suppressive drug therapies, and more, it becomes clear that it is not possible to make generalizations regarding a person's predisposition toward and expression of illness. Each case must be taken at face value, on its own terms.

Because homeopaths pay so much attention to detail, patients can find the homeopathic interview process both validating and liberating. Many come away feeling that their concerns have been truly heard for the first time. Likewise, homeopaths know that treatment will not be successful if all factors that contribute to the development of illness are not taken into account.

CHAPTER 7
Homeopathic Psychology

> *The homeopath is in the habit of studying the slightest shades of difference between patients, the little things that point to the remedy. If we looked upon disease only as the old-school physician sees it we would have no means of distinction, but it is because of the little peculiarities manifested by every individual patient, through his inner life, through everything he thinks, that the homeopath is enabled to individualize.*
>
> –James Tyler Kent, MD (1919)

One of the more unique features of homeopathy is its perspective on psychological states. We live in a culture that tends to view the majority of emotional issues as problems that must be talked out and worked out. Some can spend years in therapy, for example, trying to overcome their struggles with depression. If a problem can't be talked out, the general consensus is that the only other viable solution is drug therapy. Given this belief, it's not surprising that so many people would wind up taking psychiatric medications. Homeopathy, on the other hand, takes a very different view of such problems.

The vast majority of psychological states are temporary states that resolve with a little self-reflection, some understanding from a sympathetic ear, a cathartic release of emotion, or the passing of time. However, there are many psychological states that do not resolve, and that can eventually settle into fixed patterns. We tend to justify the persistence of such patterns of emotion and behavior as the character traits of the flawed individuals that we are.

"She's always been shy ever since she was a child." "That married man has always had a wandering eye for the ladies." "Her highly social nature makes her reluctant to be alone." "He may have a hot temper but he means well." These are the types of rationalizations that we become accustomed to when faced with having to live with such behaviors. Since there is no way to change them, we convince ourselves that they must be a normal part of life. What makes homeopathy so fascinating and satisfying is the fact that it provides a practical means by which many such undesirable behavioral and emotional patterns can be changed for the better.

A successful homeopathic prescription should yield improvements in body, mind, and spirit—literally. This is not just some slick holistic slogan or marketing ploy. It is the basis by which one judges the effects of a homeopathic medicine. Is the patient truly better in a genuine holistic sense? Does the person feel physically improved, energetically invigorated, and/or emotionally renewed? Or was there just partial relief—like the type of relief that one expects from conventional drug therapy? These are the questions that must be asked after each homeopathic prescription.

Some people, upon hearing this explanation, become concerned that homeopathy is going to change them in some undesirable way, but this is simply not the case. It is certainly true that many traits and behaviors are normal. Joe is a reserved guy, and neither he nor his friends have any problem with that. He enjoys his life and has few complaints. Susie's inhibition, on the other hand, causes her to fail to take advantage of the opportunities that come her way. It prevents her from participating fully in life. Her inhibition is a limiting mental-emotional symptom that, from a homeopathic perspective, is a function of an imbalance in the life force. Susie would not be disappointed if she could feel more socially at ease. Is a well-chosen homeopathic remedy going to turn Susie into a completely different person? No, it will not transform her into an extrovert. But it should relieve her inhibition enough to render it just a minor nuisance or a fading memory.

Even normal personality traits like independence or empathy can become limiting factors if they are exaggerated enough. One can be so independent as to be unwilling to depend upon others, always keeping life's psychological burdens to oneself. Over the years, I have seen many individuals who have become ill from an exaggerated sensitivity to others' suffering. While their empathy was admirable, it was also detrimental to their own well-being. Given enough stress in life, any trait can become a potential symptom. Good health is often a matter of balance. One can be independent while, at the same time, allowing oneself to depend upon others. One can be empathic while also maintaining healthy personal boundaries.

Bill may mean well but, when his temper starts to cause emotional distress among his family members, it becomes a problem that affects his own health and the health of those around him. Even though Bill spent the past year in counseling trying to deal with his temper, he still has a tendency to fly off the handle. This is exactly the type of issue that can be resolved with good homeopathic prescribing. It is not a problem that rises to the level of a recognized psychiatric disorder, and talk therapy has had limited impact on it. Nevertheless, homeopathic treatment can result in a world of difference for Bill and his family.

Perhaps Nancy is concerned that a homeopathic remedy will dull her ambition and desire to succeed in her chosen field of interest. After all, she says, her driven nature has allowed her to be successful. But it has also led her to the brink of burnout. I would reassure Nancy that a homeopathic remedy will not make her less successful. In fact, I expect that she will continue to be successful. But she will achieve success in a less stressed-out and more relaxed manner, in a way that will not lead to burnout and will be more conducive to her long-term health and well-being.

Homeopathic egalitarianism

Perhaps the greatest strength of homeopathy is the fact that it approaches all symptoms and conditions in democratic fashion. It takes everything presented by the patient at face value, without passing judgment as to what is relevant or not relevant. Psychological symptoms are considered just as important as physical symptoms, and sometimes more so.

Contrast this with orthodox medicine, which trains its attention almost exclusively on physical factors. Psychological influences are usually ignored even when they play indisputable roles in disease development. Not so with homeopathy, which would be rendered impotent without access to the information provided by subjective patient experience. The science referenced here in 1877 by homeopathic physician, Carroll Dunham, MD, is not conventional science. It is a more enlightened homeopathic science, one that takes into account all aspects of human illness without prejudice.

> *The eye of science regards natural phenomena with the most absolute impartiality. In her view there are no trifles, no events, subjective or objective, which are "irrelevant" and "of no moment."*[62]

Rarely is there a physical health problem that is not accompanied by a corresponding emotional state. Sometimes one can be said to cause the other, but in the majority of cases it is more complex than that. We tend to automatically assume, for example, that a person with a broken leg at the scene of a motor vehicle accident is screaming loudly *because* of the pain. This is an obvious example of cause-and-effect in the minds of most.

But then how are we to interpret the fact that different people who experience the same break in the same bone can all react quite differently? One screams in pain, another becomes angry, another cries hysterically, and yet another sits quietly in a stunned state of shock. One person maintains composure and calls for help while another rolls around, writhing in pain. Another refuses to move even an inch for fear that the pain will become worse. The one in shock attempts to get up and walk.

A broken leg is accompanied by a unique response in each case. The cause of each particular response is a function of that person, his or her health history, and the status of the vital force. Such responses, which are largely ignored by mainstream medicine, serve as vital clues for the homeopathic prescriber.

A child with an ear infection who is intensely irritable and cannot be placated requires a different homeopathic medicine than one in a weepy state desiring to be carried around by a parent. In this sense, the emotional state is not necessarily caused by the ear infection as much as it is a unique feature of the mind-body state of the child with the ear infection. Identification of such states can help lead to successful homeopathic solutions. The ear infection and state of mind are one inseparable phenomenon that must be treated as a whole.

Our psychological states, therefore, are not necessarily the logical consequences of our physical symptoms. With that said, sometimes there is a cause-and-effect relationship. In *somato-psychic* conditions, physical problems elicit emotional symptoms. In *psychosomatic* conditions, the reverse is true. In such cases, physical symptoms are the result of emotional issues and triggers. It is also possible for emotional symptoms to emerge simultaneously along with physical symptoms, as in the case of the inconsolable child with an ear infection. This is a much more common occurrence than one might think.

There is no actual separation between mind and body. Any division between the two is purely an illusion created by our indoctrination into conventional medical thinking. A single state produced by the mind-body almost always has both emotional and physical features. Symptoms tend to occur in clusters or complexes. Such patterns are not related by cause-and-effect as much as they have synchronistic relationships, which is to say that they are meaningfully related in some mysterious way that we don't fully understand. Whether emotional or physical, all symptoms are reflections of an unbalanced life force.

When psychological symptoms are understood for what they truly are, they become diagnostic clues, raw material for finding solutions to health problems. In homeopathy, it dramatically broadens the scope of what doctor and patient consider treatable. The fact that a businessman feels inadequate in the workplace but acts dictatorial towards his family at home is not just some issue that needs talking through. It is a potential clue that may help resolve his headaches and chronic indigestion. Successful treatment would be expected to help more than just his physical complaints. It should also ease his sense of inadequacy and diminish his domineering tendencies to the point of rendering them relative non-issues. Herein lies the true power and depth of homeopathy.

I believe that it is safe to say that the majority of physical illnesses can be traced to current or prior emotional disturbances. Most fail to recognize this fact because we have been programmed by material medicine and materialist culture to focus only on the physical. But homeopathy understands that the physical is inextricable from the mental-emotional and, in such cases, seeks to treat illness at its roots.

When patients discuss their main complaints, I always ask what was going on in their lives just before or at the onset of those complaints. The answers can be quite illuminating. A patient once consulted me for a variety of medically unexplained neurologic symptoms. Blood work, imaging tests, and visits to specialists had left everyone stumped. She was quite distressed over the various doctors' inability to account for her troubles.

When I asked her what was happening in her life when the symptoms began, she responded in the negative. I pressed her again, encouraging her to think about it. She welled up in tears and confessed that she had discovered that the guy she was seeing had cheated on her. Her mother had also been seriously ill around the same time. When I told her that that was plenty enough to explain why she might develop neurologic symptoms, an expression of relief came over her face. It was as if she had been given permission for the first time to own the connection between her emotions and her symptoms.

Many would agree that this is an obvious example of the type of emotional stress that can cause trouble for a lot of people. However, the majority of emotional stressors are far subtler and tend, therefore, to go unnoticed. Such stressors are the "normal" everyday events that we all experience in our lives.

Allow me to illustrate a few examples. A social clique at school leaves me out of their plans. I watch the movie, *A Nightmare on Elm Street*, and can't sleep for several nights afterwards. A friend who has forgotten our get-together stands me up. I get pushed under at the pool and swallow a mouthful of water. I proudly announce that I've gotten a raise at work but my spouse responds that the dog escaped from the yard. Someone makes a sarcastic remark about my job and later brushes it off as "just a joke." My best friend forgets my birthday. My cat gets sick and is "put to sleep." A competitor at work gets the new account instead of me. I could go on for pages, but I think you get the point.

Subtle emotional events of this nature are ubiquitous. They can be characterized as micro-traumas and, over time, they can have a cumulative effect. Even though we tend to shrug them off, they are not necessarily harmless. All people have a basic human need to be included, accepted, appreciated, respected, and loved. When those needs aren't met, it can create opportunities for illness to take root.

Remember that the life force of each individual responds differently to similar stressors. One child can feel humiliated when put on the spot by the teacher. Another doesn't care at all. A mother may take it hard when her child doesn't come home for the holidays. Her husband isn't bothered at all. Something seemingly as innocuous as the evil queen in *Snow White* can traumatize the psyche of a sensitive child. *The wounding event is in the eye of the beholder.* It is this subjective dimension of human experience that is so important to a homeopathic understanding of disease etiology.

Each person has his or her own unique Achilles heel, and the reactions to transgressions against our personal sensitivities vary greatly. A boss makes an insulting comment to his employees at work. One person shrugs it off. Another demands a meeting to clear the air. A third smolders silently in anger. A fourth takes it out on a fellow co-worker. Another turns it on himself in a fit of self-loathing. Psychological events of this sort can lay the ground for physical and emotional illness. While orthodox medicine has little use for this type of information, they serve as critical clues that lead to successful homeopathic prescriptions.

A true healer respects the diverse nature of human suffering. According to homeopathic theory, these points of vulnerability are what contribute to personal illness. When a person feels slighted by another, it makes no difference whether the allegation is true or not. From a healing perspective, the feeling of being slighted is a reality to that person, a legitimate experience that deserves to be taken seriously. In a healthier state, the same event might not have the same impact or might not even be interpreted as a slight. The fact that it is experienced as a slight is an indication that it requires attention so that it doesn't snowball into something more problematic.

The same issues can play themselves out in childrearing. From the outset, it is important to take special care of the psychological needs of children. Otherwise, wounds inflicted in childhood can grow into lifelong complexes that contribute over time to the development of chronic physical and emotional health problems.

Our lack of understanding of the unity of mind and body can lead to some mistaken ideas and unhealthy attitudes. One such attitude is the distinctly American belief that people can rise above their health problems if they really want to, especially if those problems are psychological problems. This dysfunctional cultural message suggests that people should be able overcome their emotional problems through sheer effort of will.

If this were true, then it should also be possible to exert enough willpower to overcome a hemorrhoid, a headache, or an asthma attack. Another important lesson that homeopathy teaches is that people do not willfully create their own problems. The truth is that if people were able to will themselves well, they would do so. But in most cases they don't and they can't. The sad cliché that some people just don't want to get well is a destructive notion that only adds insult to injury.

Are hypochondriacs' problems real?

Another example of the harm caused by believing that mind and body are separate entities is doctors' attitudes toward certain patients who they refer to as hypochondriacs. These are the patients who, driven by a feeling of anxiety, make frequent visits to their doctors for a variety of physical complaints.

Many such patients fall between the medical cracks when their complaints don't conform to well-defined diagnostic labels. When testing fails to reveal abnormalities, the default course of action is palliative drug treatment. When symptomatic treatment fails, these patients often wind up back in their doctors' offices begging for relief. The real issue at hand, the underlying anxiety, is never addressed.

I recall training in a family practice clinic where the names of such patients were kept in a special log. They were labeled "difficult patients." Medicine tends to view hypochondriacs as nuisances. They are complaining patients who waste doctors' time. They are generally considered malingerers who fake their symptoms. The implicit message is that their problems aren't real.

This shouldn't be surprising given the materialist orientation of medicine. Its bias is so strong that most mental, emotional, and psychological issues are treated as secondary, peripheral problems that have little to do with the "real" physical problems at hand. This mistaken notion regarding mind and body is readily apparent in the way that medicine views such patients. Once physical pathology is ruled out, there isn't much that medicine has left to offer.

Now let's contrast this with the way homeopathy views so-called hypochondriacal patients. I have seen a good number of such patients, myself. There is no doubt that their suffering is very real. Why else would they seek my assistance after having sought relief from conventional medicine many times over? Most of the time, their physical symptoms are quite real. The problem is that symptoms like anxiety, malaise, fatigue, or foggy headedness are subjective and cannot be detected or proven to exist. Fortunately, this poses no problem for a homeopath.

From a homeopathic perspective, hypochondriasis is not a convenient label that one applies to troublesome individuals. Hypochondriasis is a real and legitimate state of mind—one that requires just as much attention as an arthritic joint. It is a genuine psychological health issue.

For example, if a patient repeatedly seeks to be reassured that he or she does not have cancer in the context of a situation where there clearly is no evidence of cancer, then I must consider the possibility that it is the person's psychological state that needs my attention.

Further questioning may reveal that this individual is quite fastidious, placing a great deal of emphasis on neatness and cleanliness. There is a tendency to wake after midnight with a surge of anxiety. He also admits that he becomes cold easily and avoids consuming cold drinks. Given these clues, I might prescribe a remedy that, if successful, would be expected to relieve his anxiety about health. (Remedy choice?[63])

Another patient consults me about a number of physical complaints including fatigue, a tendency to gain weight easily, and arthritic knees. During our discussion, she mentions a concern about her mental health. It turns out that she fears developing Alzheimer's disease when she grows older. Even though she admits to no particular mental symptomatology, she brings up the topic several times during the interview.

At this point, I must consider whether her anxiety over her future mental status is a symptom that needs addressing. Further questioning reveals that she tends to perspire easily, her favorite foods include eggs and potatoes, and her arthritic knees are bothered by cold damp weather. Based on this profile, an accurate homeopathic prescription would be expected to relieve this person's fatigue, knee pain, and worry over developing Alzheimer's disease. (Remedy choice?[64])

In a conventional medical setting, such concerns would likely have been written off as something that must be tolerated when dealing with anxious patients. By contrast, there are practical homeopathic solutions for both the psychological and physical complaints. Homeopathy takes for granted that physical and emotional symptoms are equally important and equally real. Mind and body are one and therefore carry equal weight. They are one and the same.

It is misguided medical thinking to believe that mind and body can be treated separately without regard for their impact upon each other. It is even more problematic to think that the body can be treated while ignoring the distress signals of the psyche. This is one reason why conventional medicine is so prone to side effects and adverse outcomes. Suppressive treatment of physical ailments without regard for their psychic origins has a distinct tendency to drive illness deeper into the mindbody where it is more likely to manifest as mental illness.

It can be insulting for patients to be told that their psychological issues are not real, or not relevant, or all in their heads, or that they should just buck up and get over it. Conversely, it can be decidedly therapeutic to have one's emotional concerns taken seriously and given the same degree of emphasis as one's physical symptoms. It is a distinct advantage of the homeopathic approach to healing.

Mental symptoms in homeopathy

It is the standard in homeopathic circles to refer to all mental and emotional symptoms as *mentals*. Regardless of this label, there are definite differences between mental and emotional symptoms. *Emotional* symptoms involve emotions such as anger, jealousy, fear, anxiety, sadness, despair, joy, irritability, maliciousness, cowardice, impatience, and many more. Emotional symptoms are about feeling and mood. *Mental* symptoms are symptoms relating to mental functioning. They refer to dysfunctions of thought and impairment of cognitive ability. Examples of mental symptoms include confusion, poor concentration, delusions, delirium, dullness of thinking, racing thoughts, weak memory, dyslexia, difficulty reading, and so on. Although they are different, homeopaths refer to all mental and emotional symptoms as mentals.

Now there is some debate within the homeopathic community over whether a given mental should be considered a symptom or not. As

I alluded to earlier, one person may think of herself as reserved while another admits to being shy. The question, to a homeopathic practitioner, is whether a quality like reservedness is a symptom or just a normal trait, and whether it makes a difference in choosing a homeopathic remedy for that person. Some say that it should not be used as a clue if it is not seen as a problem. Others believe that such traits, even when they are not symptoms, can help identify constitutional temperament types, which can be helpful in choosing certain types of remedies.

There can be a fine line between a character trait and a symptom, and not all individuals recognize or will admit to their own dysfunctions. Such a determination involves careful judgment on the part of the prescriber. This should not be mistaken for passing judgment on the patient and his or her behavior. The intent is to use mentals as clues to help choose remedies that can assist in healing.

A mental is not necessarily considered a symptom unless it is experienced or perceived as having become stuck. Sadness, for example, can be a normal reaction to an unfortunate event. However, when it fails to release its grip and persists in spite of attempts to overcome it, the sadness may have become stuck. A push in the right direction from a dynamic energetic influence like a homeopathic medicine can relieve a great deal of unnecessary suffering in such cases.

Abandonment is a common human experience. A person may legitimately feel abandoned by friends, loved ones, or circumstances. It can be an appropriate response to real or even misunderstood events. But when a person becomes stuck in a state of feeling abandoned, that feeling can infect other relationships, even when those other relationships are on solid footing. It may eventually become the lens through which that person sees most relationships. Clearly, a feeling of abandonment is stuck when it becomes a chronic or recurring theme in a person's life. All chronic illness, for that matter, is a function of the vital force having become stuck in a negative feedback loop.

Remember that such a state, like all chronic states, reflects the life force's best way of coping with circumstances. It reflects an energetic imbalance in the life force. Oftentimes, psychotherapy is not sufficient to release a person from its hold. In such cases, it may require an energy therapy like homeopathy to restore the life force to balance.

A related issue that threatens to undermine the quality of homeopathic care is a tendency on the part of some contemporary homeopathic practitioners to overemphasize the importance of mental symptoms in case-taking and remedy selection. It is not surprising, given the psychological age we live in, that so many people would be drawn to homeopathy. After all, homeopathy recognizes the psyche's role in illness and provides a practical methodology that integrates mind and body into one exquisite system of whole person healing. As a consequence, there is a tendency for some prescribers to focus too narrowly on mental symptoms while giving insufficient attention to physical symptoms and complaints. It may be used as a shortcut to choosing a remedy that is sometimes successful but oftentimes not. Truly successful prescribing requires careful consideration of all factors, including mental, emotional, physical, medical, hereditary, and acquired factors.

People who are expecting treatment for their physical complaints may be taken aback by a homeopath's questions about their psychological status. It is an indication of how well programmed modern culture is regarding separation of mind and body. Some even feel offended when asked about their emotional tendencies and character traits. They don't understand how psychological questions could have anything to do with their physical complaints. And they don't want the doctor to think that they might have some kind of psychiatric problem. The same issue can arise when protective mothers become defensive about being asked to describe their children's behaviors. There may be tendency to paint an overly rosy picture, downplaying clues that can be useful to the homeopath. It may be necessary for the practitioner to reassure the mother about the intent of the questioning.

On the flip side, some patients can misinterpret the nature of the homeopathic interview, treating it as if it is a counseling session. A person who has never before had a doctor show interest in his or her emotional issues can understandably become overly enthusiastic, relating far more information than is necessary. There is nothing wrong with putting time aside for counseling, but the homeopathic interview shouldn't devolve into a therapy session. Overemphasis on the psychological aspects of a case can take time away from obtaining all the necessary information relating to the whole person.

Fears and delusions

Fears are a particularly important category of mental symptoms. Fears are very reliable and can point straight to certain remedies or groups of remedies. They place very prominently in the hierarchy of clues in homeopathic case analysis. By fears, I don't necessarily mean phobias. A phobia is a more extreme version of a fear. A fear doesn't have to be intense or dramatic in order for it to be a useful homeopathic clue. Of course, the more extreme a fear is, the more valuable it is in remedy selection.

Fears often go to the very heart of who we are. They say a great deal about our most vulnerable psychic points. It says a lot when a wealthy person who is financially set for life worries constantly about the possibility of poverty. The same can be said of a highly successful individual with a long track record of achievement who, nevertheless, dreads the possibility of failure.

When a person admits to having a fear of rejection, it is a good bet that the fear originates from some emotionally traumatic time in that person's life. It is also likely that the experience changed the course of that person's life, influencing important decisions along the way, and not necessarily in a positive way. Perhaps he or she backed out of a serious relationship for fear of rejection, and now regrets having made that decision. A fear of rejection can be a powerful clue that leads to the core of a case, which, in turn, can be the source of a variety of health problems.

Even common fears, like fear of heights, spiders, or thunderstorms can narrow the field of remedy choices to a significant degree. The amazing thing is that an accurate prescription not only helps the overall health of the person, it can also mitigate the intensity of the fear of that kid who refuses to sleep alone at night, or that passenger who refuses to get on the plane, or that lonely person who avoids relationships out of fear of rejection.

Some patients downplay their fears, not wanting to admit to them, or not seeing their relevance to the health problem in question. When talking about fears, a patient may say, "Isn't everyone afraid of that?" While it is true that many people are afraid of dogs, there are many more who are not. Some tend to rationalize away their fears. "I come from Australia. Why wouldn't I be afraid of snakes?" And, yet, there are many Australians who are not afraid of snakes. The fact remains that fears can say a lot about a person. They can serve as pointers that lead to a remedy, which has the potential to solve a lifetime of suffering.

Another very important category of mentals is referred to by homeopaths as *delusions*. This category is a bit different than the conventional psychiatric definition of a delusion. While there are similarities, homeopaths do not think of delusions in exactly the same way as psychiatrists. They both define a delusion as a false belief that is at odds with reality. Delusions are often maintained in the face of evidence to the contrary and in spite of common sense. Otherwise, the psychiatric and homeopathic understanding of delusions diverges widely.

In conventional psychiatry, a delusion is a sign of mental illness. Psychiatric delusions fall well outside the bounds of reality. For example, a person who, for no discernable reason, believes that the FBI is out to get him, the CIA is listening to his conversations through the radio, or an alien is watching him, is considered delusional by psychiatric standards. A delusion can be an indication of psychosis, a state in which a person has lost touch with external reality.

In homeopathy, delusions are less dramatic and far more commonplace. By homeopathic standards, delusions are false beliefs that people carry consciously or unconsciously within themselves. A delusion can dysfunctionally color the way a person sees the world and can influence the decisions he or she makes in life. While a psychotic person may believe that a terrorist has planted a bomb in his car, the homeopathic version of a delusion is subtler and less overt. A homeopathic delusion can act as a chronic stressor, exerting a negative influence on one's mental, emotional, and physical health.

I would venture to say that just about everyone labors under some type of delusional idea. For example, delusional thinking may lead a person to conclude that he or she is a failure and will never amount to anything. Some people have a distinct tendency to perceive insults where none are intended. Others think that they will never be worthy until they become the best at what they do. One person carries the distinct feeling that he is alone in life. Another feels that she is tainted in some way that makes her unlovable. These types of delusions are very common and do not rise to the level of psychiatric delusions or disorders. If they did, everyone would have a diagnosable mental illness.

Oftentimes the lines can blur. There is usually some basis in reality, some past experience that accounts for the persistence of delusional thinking. A person who has been chronically abused by a parent, for example, may carry within himself a chronic feeling of being despised. Applied to the abusive parent, it may very well be true. When that feeling of being despised extends beyond the parent-child relationship to other non-abusive relationships, then it becomes delusional thinking. In a certain sense, it doesn't really matter whether a delusional thought pattern has any basis in reality. All that matters is that it is a potentially correctable source of pain for the suffering individual.

Although it represents a perfectly understandable and very human reaction to horrific circumstances, the feeling of being despised may not objectively apply to other relationships. But it is easy to see how this type of belief can wreak havoc in a person's life. The tendency for victims of abuse to try to subconsciously work their issues out by forming relationships with other abusers is a well-documented psychological dynamic. A delusional feeling of being despised has a tendency to perpetuate the cycle of abuse. Far too often, talk therapy is not capable of dissolving the delusion.

The closer a delusional thought comes to the core of a person's being, the more significant a clue it represents to the homeopathic prescriber. When a delusional complex is deeply grafted onto the psyche, it requires strong medicine to break the bond. Nothing has the power to break the energetic spell like an accurate homeopathic prescription.

Some years back, a young man consulted me for panic attacks. It turns out he was in the midst of a spiritual crisis. Having been raised in a strongly religious family, he was met with a great deal of resistance when he tried to tell his parents that he was gay. Their response was straightforward and simple; no, he was not gay. He tried to carry on, and did so for a number of years, until he could bear the cognitive dissonance no longer.

He began to wake at night in a panic, fearful that he was being "spiritually attacked." He felt like he was being choked in his sleep. He became convinced that if he had sex with a man, "the devil will get me and I'll go crazy. God won't protect me anymore." He was taking a psychiatric drug called Zyprexa, which reduced the number of times he would wake in panic, but didn't help to resolve his issues. In order to ward off the danger, he kept his bedroom door open at night and his Bible open by his bedside. He was gripped by a fear that his sexual orientation would cost him his soul. By all other counts, this poor suffering individual was perfectly sane and in touch with reality.

Now, there happens to be a homeopathic medicine that is a good match for this man's problems. Symptoms that this substance can cause, and therefore treat, include a fear of evil, fear of going insane, and fear of demonic possession. These fears become more pronounced at night in the dark. The person that needs this remedy can exhibit compulsive behaviors and may hold the specific belief that sex is evil. I prescribed one small dose of this medicine for him to take. (Remedy choice?[65])

Two weeks later, he reported that after an initial phase of increased anxiety, he felt "better overall." The anxiety was "less intense. I don't have to leave the Bible open anymore. I'm sleeping through the night on some nights." Over the ensuing months he was instructed to take an occasional dose of the same remedy. At the three-month mark he noted, "I don't feel guilty. I accept being gay." He eventually moved out of state, was able to discontinue taking Zyprexa, has been in a long term relationship with his male partner, and has reached a point in his relationship with his parents where they accept him for who he is.

Looking back, it is clear that this young man was placed in an unbearable double bind. His sexual identity was at odds with his parents' beliefs and even his own beliefs. Something had to give, and panic, obsessive thoughts, and delusional thinking was the result. With the help of homeopathy he was able to overcome the crisis, thus enabling him to go on to live a normal, healthy life.

The vast majority of illnesses, including physical illness, can be traced to emotional sources. This basic truth is self-evident in some cases and less apparent in others. As a scientific society programmed to deny connections between the physical and the emotional, perceiving this truth is made all the more difficult. Medical interventions designed to intervene on a physiological level frequently fail to get to the root of a problem precisely because the true root is on the psychological level. This is the same reason why treatment frequently goes awry, creating unanticipated side effects and complications.

There is no denying that body and mind are one. One should not mistake this to mean that everything is in the mind. But it does mean that if a trauma or micro-trauma occurs on the emotional level, it almost always has an impact on the physical level, too. If a shocking event that causes great distress is followed weeks later by the onset of ulcerative colitis, then no amount of anti-inflammatory drug therapy alone will heal the problem. If the colitis is suppressed with powerful drugs and the emotional trauma is not properly addressed, the underlying disturbance in the life force will continue to make itself known in increasingly troublesome ways.

The mental, emotional, and energetic status of a patient is often the best indicator of overall progress. All homeopaths know that when patients truly begin to heal, they will report feeling better as a whole. They describe an overall sense of greater vitality that makes them feel like their old selves again. This can occur in spite of the persistence of physical symptomatology, which may temporarily lag behind on the healing timeline. Dr. Hahnemann, himself, described this dynamic of healing more than 200 years ago.

> *Although not visible to all, the condition of the mind, and the general behavior of the patient are among the most certain and intelligible signs of incipient improvement ... Incipient improvement, however slight, is indicated by increased sensation of comfort, greater tranquility and freedom of the mind, heightened courage, and a return of naturalness in the feelings of the patient.*[66]

When the deeper aspect of the person heals—that which may have led to the physical ailment in the first place—resolution of the physical is not far behind. As a general rule, when a homeopathic prescription results in emotional improvement, it is reasonable to expect that physical improvement will soon follow.

The truth of this healing dynamic becomes clear when we compare it to the results produced by conventional medical treatment, the stated goal of which is not intended to heal the whole person. Strong anti-arthritic drugs, for example, are often accompanied by some nasty side effects, including depression and suicidal thinking. When a patient gets relief from arthritic pain but then becomes depressed, it is not seen as a therapeutic failure as much as an unavoidable side effect to be tolerated. This, in turn, may lead to the prescription of an antidepressant. Obviously, this is not whole person healing. It is better characterized as medical whac-a-mole.

Homeopathy does not dismiss the role of mental phenomena in illness simply because it is subjective. Unhealthy emotional states are often found at the source of physical illnesses. Talk therapy can be helpful, but is usually not enough to resolve chronic dysfunctional thought patterns and the illnesses that they cause. Drug treatment can sometimes provide temporary relief but tends to lead to greater problems due to its suppressive nature. Homeopathy's advantage is that it is capable of getting to the energetic root of a problem. It understands the role of the psyche in illness and strives to heal each unique illness, mentally, emotionally, and physically, from inside out.

CHAPTER 8

The True Nature of Health and Healing

> *If the removal of symptoms is not followed by a restoration to health, it cannot be called a cure.*
> –James Tyler Kent, MD (1919)

> *Vital to developing the homeopathic vision is the understanding of what is to be cured in disease. It is to be able to perceive, to feel and to know as the truth that disease is not something local but a disturbance of the whole being. It is to have the unshakable conviction that if we treat the disturbance at the centre, the local problems will be lessened.*
> –Rajan Sankaran, MD (1992)

When you think about it, there is something conspicuously absent from conventional medical discourse. We hear a great deal about new diagnostic technologies. We hear about the latest drugs on the market, warnings of the side effects that come with them, and scientific studies that justify their use. Then we hear about the latest research, which not infrequently contradicts previous research. But there is one particular topic that we never hear about, that the medical establishment won't touch with a ten-foot pole. There is no serious discussion about what it means to be healthy—or to be sick for that matter.

The topic gets little attention from the medical establishment, which is too busy conducting "science" to stop and contemplate larger issues that could provide a roadmap to guide that science. Without a roadmap, science wanders here and there, wasting tremendous resources pursuing one dead end after another. It often appears that medicine has no compass at all. This lack of guiding principles makes medicine easy prey to outside influences. As a result, it has strayed far from its original mission of healing the sick.

The foundation of homeopathic healing, on the other hand, is built upon a clearly thought-out conception of the nature of health and illness. The pioneers of homeopathy felt it important enough to write entire books on the topic of homeopathic principles and philosophy. Homeopathic philosophy is indispensible to the science and practice of homeopathic medicine. Principles of healing guide the practice of homeopathy, just as the lessons learned from treating patients help to clarify and sharpen those homeopathic principles.

So what are those principles of healing and how were they formulated? As previously noted, it began with Dr. Hahnemann who discovered a practical means to apply the principle of similars. Prior to Hahnemann, the concept had been contemplated by the likes of Paracelsus and Hippocrates, but largely on theoretical grounds. Hahnemann found a consistent way to put his principle into action for a wide range of health conditions. Hahnemann's observations led him to conclude that the principle of similars was a more effective method than the prevailing treatments of the time, which employed the use of opposites to combat symptoms. Treatment by opposites remains the dominant approach in medicine to this day.

Hahnemann's successors contributed a great deal to his revolutionary system of healing. One particularly important contributor was Constantine Hering, MD, who formulated a principle referred to by contemporary homeopaths as Hering's Law. There is a great deal of discussion about whether Hering's Law should be considered an actual law of healing, or whether Dr. Hering was even the author of the law attributed to his name.[67] I'll let the historians haggle over the details but, suffice it to say, Hering's Law illustrates several very important principles of healing. One might say that Hering's Law is the yardstick by which one judges whether or not a treatment is truly effective.

However, before we can ponder over principles of healing, we must first define what it is that constitutes good health. Judging one's state of health from a homeopathic perspective is completely different than judging health according to allopathic standards. Or should I say, a homeopathic assessment involves much more than the criteria used by conventional medicine. Evaluating health by objective measures like a physical exam and lab values is just the tip of the iceberg. A homeopathic assessment goes much further because it includes the subjective dimension of health. A person's own sense of health, well-being, vitality, and emotional balance are taken very seriously.

It is not possible to reduce good health to a simplistic slogan like "health is the absence of dis-ease" Is it sufficient to judge health by the presence or absence of symptoms? Is a person healthy if blood work and a physical exam reveal nothing of concern? Perhaps such criteria are good enough for conventional medical purposes, but they are too vague to meet homeopathic standards. Does the absence of a conventional diagnosis constitute good health? Certainly these criteria by themselves are not sufficient. Many a person who has been given a clean bill of conventional medical health continues, nevertheless, to feel unwell.

In defining health we are immediately confronted by the materialistic and objectivist limitations of conventional medicine. Good health to the conventional physician means good *physical* health. Orthodox medicine takes into account mental and emotional health only in the most superficial of ways. If a patient complains of being too easily bothered by stories of suffering individuals, or is prone to jealousy, or confesses to feeling insecure, or tends to be disorganized, there is little that orthodox medicine can do. While such intangible complaints are too subjective for medical science, they fall directly into the wheelhouse of homeopathic practice.

From a broader homeopathic perspective, the notion of symptomatology takes on a whole new meaning. By this standard, a child's fear of spiders and an adult's reluctance to deal with situations that involve potential conflict are symptomatic indicators of less than ideal health. They are also diagnostic clues that can help solve homeopathic cases.

The homeopathic definition of health, therefore, is far more inclusive. Homeopathy takes into account emotional, mental, spiritual, *and* physical health. Good health constitutes the absence of limiting symptoms on all levels. Note here my use of the term *limiting*. It is not realistic to define health as a complete absence of symptoms. Symptoms serve a legitimate purpose. They are, by definition, adaptive responses of the life force to a variety of stressors. The question is whether the life force is capable of rebounding quickly back to a state of balance. Adaptive symptoms should be transitory phenomena. When they persist, symptoms become limiting factors. They signify a life force that has been thrown off balance.

Whether an emotion like jealousy is considered a symptom or not depends upon various factors, including its frequency, intensity, and the degree to which it interferes with a person's ability to function in life and in relationships. If a fear of water prevents one from learning how to swim, then it is a problem that can benefit from treatment. Any personal issue that deprives one of the ability to make choices in life can, therefore, be considered an impediment to ideal health.

From an energetic perspective, homeopathic theory posits that true health depends upon the health of the vital force. A healthy life force is capable of adapting to life's circumstances without becoming compromised. Persistent symptoms are signs that the life force has become stuck, unable to flow freely. Energy that is blocked or impeded or trapped in a bottleneck produces symptoms that can be expressed on physical, emotional, mental, or spiritual levels.

Of course, making judgments about the health of an individual and his or her physical, emotional, mental, and spiritual status requires maturity, experience, and discernment. It is a great responsibility that often requires the practitioner to "read between the lines" in order to identify problems or issues that the patient may not necessarily be willing to discuss openly and frankly. It requires sensitivity, compassion, an ability to communicate effectively, and an awareness of one's own personal issues, which, if not taken into account, can have a tendency to cloud one's judgment.

Given the fact that a high percentage of physical ailments can be traced back to emotional distress and/or faulty thinking, it becomes clear how critical it is to be versed in the nature of the psyche and its relationship to the human body. In this sense, personal growth should be the mission of all homeopathic practitioners. Life itself becomes the training ground that provides the necessary wisdom and experience to be the most effective healer that one can be.

Health is not a static state that one should seek to preserve. It is an organic process that flows with life's twists and turns. The moment the life force gets stuck and ceases to flow is the moment when pathology begins to take root. Healing, therefore, is a process that also takes twists and turns. And, as all homeopaths will tell you, there are principles that can guide us, that tell us whether the healing process is proceeding in the correct direction. It can be said that disease moves in a direction opposite to healing. I discuss this "directionality of disease" at some length in my book, *Green Medicine*.[68] By the same token, there is a directionality to healing. It is important to understand how real healing takes place, and this brings us back to the topic mentioned earlier—Hering's Law.

Basic principles of healing

So what is Hering's Law and why is it so important? It can be summed up by the following ideas:

- Genuine healing takes place from inside out, from interior to exterior, from deeper to more superficial aspects of the whole person.
- Genuine healing moves from the center to the periphery, from more vital to less vital organs and parts of the body.
- Genuine healing tends to take place from above downward, from the head down to the toes.
- Genuine healing occurs from present to past as the life force retraces its steps by manifesting symptoms in approximately the reverse order from how they originally occurred.

In essence, healing takes place from inside out, from top to bottom, and from present to past. Hering's so-called Law should not be taken too literally, not in the sense of a law that cannot be broken. It is preferable to think of Hering's Law as a flexible set of guiding principles. When the trajectory of a person's health follows one or more of these principles, it is a good sign that healing is moving in the correct direction. Let's take a look at some practical examples:

Example 1

A person with depression and suicidal thinking receives a homeopathic prescription of *Natrum sulphuricum*. One month later at the return visit, he reports feeling significant relief from depression and an absence of suicidal thoughts. He also notes that soon after taking the remedy he developed a head cold that lasted for two weeks. The cold manifested mainly as head congestion and a profusely runny nose.

This is a straightforward illustration of Hering's principle that healing takes place from inside out. The deeper emotional state improved while less threatening and more superficial cold symptoms took its place. The illness moved from the deeper mental plane to the physical level. In a sense, the cold symptoms served as an outlet, a safe avenue for healing.

It should be noted that many healing responses take the form of bodily discharges like the runny nose in this example. All homeopaths know that it is not wise to artificially thwart a discharge with suppressive drug therapies. The consequences can be less than desirable.

Example 2

A woman having painful gallbladder attacks is given several doses of *Chelidonium*. As the attacks fade away, she develops pain in her right shoulder, which lasts for several weeks.

This example illustrates Hering's observation that healing occurs from the center to the periphery, from more vital to less vital parts of the body. In this case, the focal point of the disturbance in the life force moves from a deeper internal organ to a less dangerous pain in the shoulder.

We, as a society, have been programed to want instant gratification. We expect immediate relief from our health complaints, too. It can be tricky business to convince a person to wait through weeks of shoulder pain in order to allow the life force the time it needs to heal itself from a deeper gall bladder problem. Some are unwilling to wait. If this woman were to succumb to the desire for painkilling medication, the suppressive nature of drug therapy would increase the likelihood of the return of her gallbladder attacks.

I recall treating a woman with severe gallbladder attacks who called me from a local hospital. She was admitted on a Friday but had to wait until Monday to undergo surgery to remove her gallbladder. I prescribed one strong dose of *Lycopodium*. She called back that weekend to report that her pain was dramatically improved. With concern in her voice, she noted that she had also voided a large quantity of urine with a distinctly orange color. I explained that it was most likely a healing discharge. It was her body's way of rechanneling the disturbance away from the gallbladder. Come Monday, she refused surgery and convinced the surgeon to discharge her from the hospital. I've known her for years; she's never had a gallbladder problem since.

Example 3

During medical school, the doctor who taught me homeopathy consulted on a particularly severe and chronic case of eczema that covered much of a patient's body. This patient was the brother of my friend, who also happened to be a fellow medical student. As a consequence, I was given frequent reports on his brother's progress. He was prescribed doses of *Natrum muriaticum* on a bi-weekly basis. To my friend's astonishment, with each dose the eczema would begin to recede from the arms and upper half of his brother's body. Gradually, the eczema retreated to the lower portions of his legs. After months of treatment, a horrific case of eczema had become a mere nuisance in this young man's life.

Of course, this is an illustration of the principle that healing takes place from above downward. Although I have witnessed this phenomenon a good number of times, this is perhaps the least reliable aspect of Hering's Law. Nevertheless, when it does occur, it is a good sign that genuine healing is under way.

Example 4

A woman of menopausal age complains of a general lack of energy, an unexplained dissatisfaction with her family life, and a growing aversion to sexual intimacy with her husband. Her past history includes a variety of menstrual complaints, long-standing birth control use prior to her having children, and episodes of right sided sciatica when she was in her thirties. She is prescribed two doses of a homeopathic medicine (Remedy choice?[69])

Four weeks later, she reports general improvement in her energy and mood. She acknowledges feeling more physically attracted to her husband. She also notes that twice she began to bleed and was convinced that she was about to get her period, which she had not had in over six months. In between the two bleeding episodes, she experienced a surprising blast from the past. It was a flare-up of sciatica, which turned out to be mild and relatively short lived compared to past flare-ups.

Here we have an illustration of the way in which healing occurs from present to past. In this case, the most recent state of poor energy and emotional dissatisfaction is exchanged for brief recurrences of older hormonal dysfunction and sciatic pain. The life force can be said to be retracing its steps as it winds its way back to a better state of overall health.

Only a small percentage of those familiar with homeopathy truly understand Hering's Law. Most patients receiving homeopathic care do not recognize these principles of healing, even when they experience them firsthand. They don't take conscious note of how it happens. This makes it all the more important to educate the public about what real healing looks like and how it actually takes place. Good health is not something that can be judged by whether or not one is sick at the present moment. Health is a state that is subject to change and healing is a process that takes place over time. Either one is moving in a positive healing direction—the direction of cure—in accordance with Hering's Laws, or one is not.

The alternative is the standard by which most people judge health—the conventional medical status quo. But do we really understand what happens when we employ allopathic methods of treatment? Are we fully aware of the short and long-term consequences? I would contend that most people are not. Most people are just happy to find that their symptoms have gone away. They tend not to look at the larger picture and the connections between one illness and the next, and the next. If they did, they might be surprised by the patterns they notice.

Just as there is a direction of healing, so, too, there is directionality to disease. But mainstream medical culture prevents us from becoming aware of it. We are conditioned not to connect the dots. Perhaps it is more accurate to say that even the medical establishment does not connect the dots. Because if it did, it would precipitate a crisis of conscience and a crisis of care.

When we pay closer attention, however, the directionality of disease becomes easily discernable. It simply requires that we connect the dots between one medical event and the next. Allow me to illustrate with a few more examples that *do* connect the dots.

Example 5

A child with an ear infection is treated with a standard course of antibiotics. He recovers after about a week, but continues to have a poor appetite, which persists for another week. Six weeks later, he develops another infection in the same ear. Antibiotics are prescribed, the infection clears up, and this time his lack of appetite persists for several more weeks. By the time a year has passed, the child has endured six ear infections, each one requiring an antibiotic. His picky appetite has become chronic and the range of foods that he will eat has steadily narrowed.

This is an example of a fairly common pattern. Clearly something is amiss here. Is it fair to say that each ear infection was a separate and discreet medical event, and that each course of antibiotics "cured" each individual ear infection? Is it possible that antibiotic treatment somehow contributed to the chronicity of this child's ear infections? Why would a physician pursue a course of action like this knowing that it contributes to a vicious cycle of chronicity?

From a homeopathic perspective, this represents one single ongoing state of ill health that is not responding to treatment. At best, it can be characterized as palliation in the sense that the child experiences temporary relief with each course of antibiotics. It is even debatable whether the antibiotics were helping at all. Research has shown that kids with ear infections tend to get better regardless of whether they take antibiotics or not. Alternately, this can be seen as an example of suppression, wherein drug therapy appears to solve one problem while leading to another more chronic problem. What started as a single ear infection has morphed into a case of recurrent ear infections and chronic poor appetite.

Example 6

A woman has a painful shoulder that does not respond well to physical therapy. Her physician recommends a cortisone injection. The relief is almost instantaneous and she is pain-free for six months. When the pain returns to the same shoulder, another cortisone shot brings relief but, this time, it is of shorter duration. Surprisingly, she begins to experience pain in the other shoulder. A cortisone shot is administered to that shoulder, too. To make a long story short, two years later, the same woman has chronic pain in both her shoulders and knees. She has been diagnosed with arthritis and takes anti-inflammatory drugs on a daily basis to manage the pain.

Most conventional physicians would attribute the spread of this woman's arthritis to the idea that it was not "caught" on time. They would argue that had more aggressive treatment been instituted earlier, the outcome might have been more favorable. This is a good example of medical rationalism. Medicine adjusts its theories and alters its logic to suit its needs. This particular explanation saves face and preserves the integrity of the practice of using cortisone injections for painful joints.

From a homeopathic perspective this represents a classic case of suppression. The treatment is responsible for the spread of the illness. Even mainstream medicine acknowledges that cortisone is an immunosuppressive drug. It suppresses the body's immune response. In this case, it prevents the body from attacking its own tissues. The problem is that it only does so temporarily. It creates a false appearance of cure by driving the disease deeper, in this case encouraging the spread of arthritis to new locations. Had it been left alone from the start, the arthritis might have been confined to its original location. Suppressive measures increase the likelihood that it will spread, making it much harder to treat in the long run.

Example 7

A woman with asymptomatic hepatitis C under my homeopathic care decided one day to try a new drug that was advertised as being able to "cure" her condition. As a result of treatment her viral load became undetectable. In other words, testing no longer found any evidence of hepatitis C in her body. Over the years, she had occasionally mentioned having minor pain in her hands, but nothing of consequence. It would come and go but never caused her to seek treatment. However, after taking the new hepatitis drug the pain escalated rapidly and did not abate. Her fingers became visibly deformed.

Here we have another case of suppression. The forcible pharmaceutical suppression of this woman's viral hepatitis titer has resulted in the acceleration of a previously mild and inconsequential arthritic condition of her hands. As is typical in many cases of suppression, conventional medicine denies the connections, writing them off to coincidence. In the case of this new drug, the so-called cure is measured by improving lab values while conveniently ignoring the drug's impact upon the whole person. This patient started with abnormal lab values but no symptoms and wound up with normal lab values and chronic pain.

Example 8

A young boy has seasonal allergies. His symptoms are managed with a variety of drugs including antihistamines and steroid-based nasal sprays. From one year to the next the allergy symptoms gradually diminish, but during that same time frame he begins to have trouble breathing. His new diagnosis of asthma is treated with additional drugs including stronger doses of steroids. After adjusting his drug regimen, the asthma becomes more manageable. However, his teachers notice that he now has difficulty focusing in school. He is having trouble sleeping and his parents report that he has become irritable at home. Recently, he threw several temper tantrums, which is unusual for him. His parents take him to a psychiatrist, concerned that their son may have attention deficit disorder.

This type of scenario has become a routine occurrence in modern life. Many thousands of kids are afflicted with allergies, asthma, and attention deficit problems. The numbers are skyrocketing but no one knows why. Or should I say that no one wants to connect the dots because it might force them to acknowledge the elephant in the room. The only mystery here is the collective denial of the medical establishment.

Most homeopaths can identify the source of this boy's problems quite easily. The original allergy symptoms were subdued with suppressive treatments, thus driving the illness deeper, causing the life force to manifest the disturbance as asthma instead. Similarly suppressive drugs aimed at the asthma further weaken the life force, driving the problem even deeper until it finally metastasizes to the mental-emotional plane, thereby generating symptoms that resemble attention deficit disorder.

While examples 1 through 4 demonstrate the direction of healing, examples 5 through 8 are illustrations of the directionality of disease. All cases highlight the idea that health and illness are not static phenomena—they are ongoing lifelong processes. One's state of health can be said to be moving either in a positive or negative direction, toward greater health and vitality or toward more compromising health issues.

It is easy to lose track of the overall direction of healing when we focus our attention only on the most immediate symptoms and local problems. It behooves us to take a step back to survey the entire situation in order to assess the cumulative impact of all problems that impinge upon the person as a whole. We employ tunnel vision when we declare eczema cured because it has disappeared after applying a prescription cream. When eczema fades away only to be replaced a few weeks later by frequent stomachaches, then we must question whether it was cured or suppressed.

If the medical establishment opened its eyes to such trends and the general public was educated about these issues, it would make a significant difference in how we approach health and illness. If society became cognizant of the differences between the direction of healing and the directionality of disease, which do you think it would choose? While it may be pie-in-the-sky thinking, we do have to start somewhere. This is one reason for my writing this book.

A great deal of chronic illness in the modern world is triggered and maintained by suppressive drug therapies. Homeopathy is comparatively safe, does not contribute to chronic disease, and is capable of reversing the directionality of disease. Homeopathy can assist the vital force in turning the tide in favor of true healing, toward the direction of cure.

About terminology

It should be understood that there are important differences between *treatment, healing, cure, suppression,* and *palliation*. Conventional medicine frequently and inappropriately interchanges these terms with little awareness of their true meanings. For the sake of clarity, I will briefly discuss the differences here.

As we have said, *healing* and *disease* are processes that change over time. One moves in a positive direction, the other in a negative direction—the wrong direction. *Suppression* is brought about by outside interventions that unnaturally force matters toward the direction of disease.

Cure is a theoretical endpoint, an ideal of perfect health that is never technically reached. There is always some health issue or weakness in the vital force that can benefit from proper care. For this reason, in my opinion it is not wise to speak of curing illness. When orthodox medicine speaks of cure, it is referring to suppression of specific symptoms or illnesses. Allopathic cure is a reductionist construct that fails to take into account the larger picture. When health is moving in a positive direction, rather than refer to it as *cure*, I believe it is preferable to use the terms *healing* or *improving health*.

Truth be told, I dislike the word *cure* even in the context of homeopathy. The homeopathic literature is filled with frequent references to *cured cases* and *incurable diseases*. I dislike both terms because they imply a degree of certainty and finality that is not warranted. Both represent prognostic overreach.

Palliation occurs when a drug temporarily causes symptoms to improve. It is expected that they will return at a later point. *Palliation* brings short-term relief followed by a return of symptoms. *Suppression* occurs when a drug forcibly causes symptoms to completely disappear—or at least enough to create new problems. The vast majority of pharmaceuticals act by suppressing and/or palliating symptoms. The suppressive and palliative actions of drugs are what give allopathic medicine its razzle-dazzle. Those who are impressed by the illusion of short-term allopathic "cures" often wind up disappointed in the long run.

Treatment is a neutral term that implies nothing specific regarding outcomes. Treatment can result in healing, palliation, suppression, or nothing at all. *Management* is another term commonly used in medicine. The management of an illness implies that it can only be contained at best, and that healing and cure are not to be expected.

Sometimes palliation is necessary as in the case of an asthma attack that requires an inhaler to keep a person safe. Although it is best to avoid suppression if possible, it is not predictable whether palliative treatment will bring temporary relief or lead to permanent suppression. Suffice it to say that the medical establishment commonly misuses all of the aforementioned terms.

It should be clear that there is no such thing as a perfect state of health. Perfect health will always remain just an ideal. The pursuit of better health is an ongoing process that, arguably, will continue into the next lifetime and the one after that. There are many who believe that symptoms are necessary for growth. They provide the incentive that allows us to move beyond our previous limitations. There is always room for psychological growth, greater maturity, deeper spiritual understanding, and evolution of consciousness.

A healing crisis by any other name

Any good book about homeopathy inevitably comes round to a discussion of the concept of the homeopathic *aggravation*. Patients are told that their symptoms may temporarily worsen before they get better. And this is true. An accurate prescription has a tendency to stir things up a bit before improvement takes place.

I tell my patients that there is a possibility that the remedy will cause a flare-up of something before their condition improves. What that something will be I cannot say. Sometimes their main complaint will act up. A person seeking help for migraines may develop a migraine or a person with an arthritic knee may have a flare of knee pain. Sometimes it's something seemingly unrelated to the main complaint. It could be a head cold, or a fever, or an allergy attack, or a skin rash, or a sudden attack of sleepiness, or a fit of temper, or a crying jag. You name it—it's a possibility.

A homeopathic aggravation usually happens within hours or days of taking the *simillimum*—sometimes even minutes. It may last minutes, hours, or a few days, but not much longer than that. Sometimes there is no aggravation at all. Sometimes the reaction is mild; sometimes it's stronger than that. The important thing to realize is that an aggravation is a manifestation of the vital force's efforts to heal itself.

Oftentimes, something unusual happens in the midst of, or as a consequence of an aggravation. The person seeking help for asthma comes down with a cold but also notes with surprise that it did not trigger an asthma attack like it typically does. A person with recurrent dreams of being chased has another dream, but this time he turns around to confront his pursuer. Another person develops a fever that comes and goes within a matter of hours. I have learned not to be surprised by such events.

An aggravation is the very same phenomenon referred to by a variety of holistic practitioners as a *healing crisis*. The term sounds rather dramatic and can be a little alarming to the uninitiated. Even the word "aggravation" can cause some patients to balk when it comes time to take their homeopathic prescription. I have had some patients tell me that they will take the remedy at the end of their workweek, only to have them call weeks later to reschedule their follow-up appointment because they have still not taken the remedy. Some never do.

For this reason, I gently explain the idea of a homeopathic aggravation to my patients so as not to provoke anxiety. Although homeopathy is extremely safe, it is nevertheless a very powerful therapy. I tell my patients that the reason I practice homeopathy is because I could not bring myself to practice conventional medicine given its side effects and dangers. The risks of conventional drugs are far greater. When an aggravation of symptoms does take place, it is usually a good sign. It is well worth putting up with the temporary discomfort in order to reap the benefits.

It is not possible to predict with any accuracy the specific nature of a homeopathic aggravation. Every situation is different and each individual will respond differently in accordance with the uniqueness of his or her symptomatic circumstances. Ten individuals given the same remedy in the same potency will all respond in different ways, ways that could not have been anticipated. One thing is clear though; it will not bring them harm.

Another important point, which can be hard to convey, is that an aggravation is definitely not the same thing as a side effect. Side effects are symptoms that patients must endure while taking conventional medications. They must be tolerated, sometimes indefinitely, as long as one wishes to be the recipient of the so-called benefits of a medication. The term, *side effects*, is a euphemism designed to downplay the reality that they are, in fact, the *direct* but unwanted effects of a drug. They are referred to as side effects in order to minimize their psychological impact, thus ensuring that patients don't refuse to take their prescriptions.

By contrast, an aggravation is a temporary and desirable effect of a homeopathic prescription. It is a sign that the remedy is beginning to work. An aggravation is the beginning of a transition phase between the current state of illness and a future state of improved health and vitality. It is an indication that the vital force is responding to the stimulus represented by the homeopathic medicine. Before order can be restored, a certain amount of upheaval may have to take place. An aggravation can be understood as the life force's attempt to break free from its previous pattern of ill health. It is an attempt to alter the status quo by shifting the balance from certain symptoms to other, less threatening symptoms.

Once an aggravation takes place, all that remains is to sit back and observe whether it produces subsequent signs of improving health. Sometimes it appears to help, only to fizzle out over time, in which case another dose may be required or a different medicine may be indicated. Oftentimes, positive changes can persist for weeks or even months; hence the need to be patient once improvements are noticed.

It is possible in some cases to minimize the intensity and/or duration of an aggravation by carefully choosing the appropriate dose of the indicated remedy. This is a complicated topic that generates a great deal of debate within the homeopathic community. There are disagreements over potency and even disagreements over the value and necessity of homeopathic aggravations. The bottom line is that unlike side effects, aggravations do not cause harm. An aggravation is an indication that the life force is responding to the homeopathic prescription.

The time factor

A common myth is that it takes a long time for homeopathy to work. Nothing could be further from the truth. It is true, however, that it may take some time for the prescriber to determine the correct homeopathic medicine.

The search for the *simillimum* (the one medicine that best fits the case) can be a trial and error process. If the prescribed remedy does not help, then another medicine must be chosen. This process continues until the *simillimum* is found. Only in this sense does homeopathy take time to work. Once the correct medicine is taken, improvement is usually rapid and sometimes even dramatic.

Conventional medicine has an advantage in that most medications need to be taken on a daily basis. This has the net effect of appeasing unhappy patients who might otherwise be right back in the doctor's office demanding relief from their suffering. Patients are often told that it may take weeks before the effects of their medicines kick in. A daily dose can serve as a placebo that keeps patients from giving up on their allopathic treatment.

Many homeopaths, on the other hand, prescribe just a single or a few doses, after which the patient is expected to wait a number of weeks in order to determine the full impact of the remedy. This, of course, is the case when dealing with chronic illnesses. When treating an acute illness, like an ear infection for example, the waiting time is by necessity much shorter.

Orthodox medicine has no concept of healing as a process that takes place over the course of time. And it has no expectation of healing in the sense that a homeopath thinks of healing. When a person has migraines, a painkiller is usually prescribed. That is the extent of the conventional medical thought process regarding migraines. It is assumed that migraines will continue to recur.

The purpose of homeopathic treatment would be to eliminate the migraines completely by restoring balance to the life force. The process of rebuilding a person's health from the ground up can, admittedly, take some time—but it is well worth the time invested. It is certainly preferable to a passive state of resignation that assumes migraines will remain a long-term companion.

The process of restoring a person's health and vitality varies greatly depending upon a multitude of factors including past health history and current health status. It is not unusual to see, for example, a patient who had eczema and multiple ear infections as a child, asthma and a sports-related concussion as an adolescent, and depression and hypertension as an adult. It only makes sense that it can take time and effort to rebuild such a person's health, especially in light of the fact that orthodox medicine has no such ability to do the same.

Remember that a homeopath views health and illness as ongoing lifelong processes. Think of the patient's eczema and ear infections as steppingstones that led eventually to asthma. Add to that a concussion and all those factors together combine to render the patient susceptible to depression and hypertension. Conventional medicine does not acknowledge this larger perspective because it has no means by which to reverse such trends. The best it can do is focus its attention on the current problem at hand, which, in this example, would be the depression and hypertension.

A timeline is an indispensible tool because it allows the homeopathic practitioner to arrange a person's health-related life events in chronological order. It makes it possible to visualize the layers of a case or the pieces of the puzzle so to speak. The peeling away of the layers of an onion is an apt metaphor for the homeopathic healing process. This is exactly what happens when the vital force reacts positively to a well-chosen homeopathic remedy.

If, for example, a person with a history of a concussion fifteen years earlier seeks help for his current state of fatigue and depression, it would not be surprising to find that as he improves he goes through a brief phase of headaches that reminds him of his old post-concussion recovery period.

Another patient seeks homeopathic treatment for chronic symptoms related to recurrent sinus infections. She complains of a great deal of post-nasal mucus production. The mucus is very thick, yellow, and stringy. The nose is chronically stuffed up, producing a nasal quality to her voice. The mornings are spent coughing up mucus that has accumulated in the respiratory passages overnight. (Remedy choice?[70])

When she returns she notes that all symptoms have vanished and her sinuses have cleared, but she now reports that her left leg is aching. One can be reassured that this is the direction of healing when it is discovered that, according to a timeline of her health history, she had an episode of left-sided sciatica ten years prior. It serves as further confirmation when she notes that the ache is reminiscent of the old sciatica.

Sadly, stories of physical, psychological, and sexual abuse are commonplace among patients who seek my care. Many believe that they have moved past those old traumas, while others have managed to block out or forget the memories and feelings associated with their past. While these may be useful survival mechanisms that can help people to cope, it does not necessarily mean that they have healed from these terrible events. Unbeknownst to most, the scars of old traumas can continue to generate symptoms, even many years later. Some complain of headaches and fatigue, some can't think or concentrate, while others struggle with fibromyalgia or sleep disorders. The possibilities are endless.

When a person with a history of past psychological trauma undergoes homeopathic treatment for their current symptoms, it would be surprising if old emotions relating to that trauma did not make an appearance. As the fatigue or headaches or body aches begin to resolve, old unresolved psychological issues can emerge to take their place.

On occasion, a patient may experience a panic attack during the course of treatment. Panic in such a case is not necessarily a negative thing. It is usually the consequence of a surge of unidentified emotion that has been long buried and is now trying to make its way to the surface. At first those emotions threaten to overwhelm the psyche—hence the feeling of panic—but eventually, as those emotions are identified and the memories attached to them are recalled, the panic begins to fade away. The road to deep, lasting, and genuine healing is well on its way.

In the examples above, the sciatica and panic attacks represent the emergence of old layers. This is made possible thanks to the space created by the resolution of more recent problems. As one problem fades, it makes room for the next layer to surface once again. This is a common experience for patients undergoing homeopathic treatment. Some are puzzled when such events occur. They may believe that they had "dealt" with a particular problem and are understandably surprised when it resurfaces. Its reemergence is evidence that it never did fully resolve and may have been contributing to the chronicity of current health problems.

Every case is unique. No one health timeline is like any other and the status of the vital force varies greatly from person to person. Old pieces to the health puzzle can take many forms. Injuries like broken bones and strained back muscles, illnesses like the flu, pneumonia, and mononucleosis, and traumas like car accidents, frightening experiences, and psychological and sexual abuse represent just a few. Even energetically inherited issues from past generations can contribute layers to a case. Medical treatment, itself, is a significant factor that can create new layers in a person's health history. Each suppressive drug taken and every surgery endured is a potential seed from which new problems can grow.

Not all such events leave scars but some represent potential obstacles that may resurface during treatment and must be overcome on the road back to genuine health. Due to the unique nature of each case, it is not possible to predict the course of events with any accuracy. Each case must be met on its own terms as events unfold. There are no shortcuts and no predetermined protocols to make the job easier. Likewise, there is no way to tell how long the healing process will take. It is up to the life force, which determines the pace and course of events.

Since the life force dictates the pace of healing, it is not desirable to speed the process up artificially. Attempts to do so by repeating remedies when they are not needed can sometimes backfire, thus prolonging the recovery process. One can only assist the process by supporting the life force's efforts to heal itself.

Orthodox medicine has neither the patience for such a process nor any understanding of how it works. It contents itself, instead, with suppressive measure after suppressive measure, which creates a false impression of healing. The net effect tends to be a gradual decline in the strength, resilience, and vitality of the life force.

True healing requires patience and perseverance. This is the nature of genuinely individualized medical care. Homeopathy, when practiced correctly, does just that.

Treating symptoms versus healing the whole person
It should be clear by now that orthodox medicine takes a targeted approach to illness. It focuses almost exclusively on the most immediate and local physical problems. Its seeks to eliminate the most pressing symptoms at the present moment. It promises little regarding overall health or long-term well-being.

When a person with an inflamed gallbladder seeks orthodox care, doctors have only the expectation that surgery will remove the patient from immediate danger. There is no consideration for longer-term implications. It is not uncommon for such a patient to continue to complain of digestive discomfort, even after surgery. Regardless of whether the patient also complains of fatigue, diarrhea, and irritability, those issues are of little concern to the surgeon who considers the job done once the gallbladder has been removed and the patient is no longer in immediate danger.

You might ask, what's wrong with that? Isn't that what surgery is supposed to accomplish? And the answer is, yes, that is what we have been conditioned to expect from a system of medicine that claims to have the only answers to such problems. However, from a homeopathic perspective, there is much more that can be done. It is reasonable to think that the gallbladder can be saved, digestive normalcy can be restored, and long-term well-being can be maximized.

In this sense, Western medicine has very little to do with true healing. Its concept of healing is more like convalescing after surgery or lying in bed recovering from pneumonia. I'm not knocking the fact that medicine is this way. Conventional medicine is ideal for emergencies and late-stage illnesses after all other options have been exhausted. But it should not be mistaken for real healing. That would be an awfully low bar to set.

Not infrequently, I find myself having to answer the question, "What is this remedy supposed to do, doc?" Clearly, patients want to know how the medicines work. Do they stop inflammation? Do they lower blood pressure? Do they kill viruses? In other words, patients want to know the mechanisms of action behind homeopathic medicines. They ask because they have become accustomed to a medical system that provides lots of explanations but few real solutions.

Trying to answer such questions can be like trying to communicate with someone in a foreign language. When I explain that a homeopathic prescription is not designed to target the main complaint as much as it is aimed at healing the whole person, it tends to elicit more questions. If I claim that homeopathy can help a person avoid surgery, end gallbladder pain, and relieve fatigue, diarrhea, and irritability, I am likely to meet with skepticism. Nevertheless, I have seen such results more than a few times in my homeopathic career.

To answer the question honestly, a good homeopathic prescription restores balance to an out-of-balance life force. It does not target any specific symptom. It does not act through any identifiable physiological mechanism. It is neither a painkiller nor an antibiotic. While it may be true that a well-chosen remedy can relieve pain, reduce inflammation, and restore proper physiologic functioning, it does not do so directly. It does so by restoring the whole person to a state of bioenergetic balance. When the life force re-establishes balance, symptoms become no longer necessary.

Such an answer can frustrate people who think in conventional medical terms. For some, it may seem like a gimmicky, made-up, New Agey answer. But it is the best answer that I have to offer. It is an answer designed to explain how homeopathic medicines can have such long-lasting and far-reaching effects. Such effects cannot be explained via reductionist thinking. They can only be understood from a holistic perspective. It is an answer that explains a repeatedly observed phenomenon that defies the boundaries of conventional scientific thought.

Successful homeopathic treatment should result in restoration of health, not just the elimination of symptoms. Restoration of health means the vital force is free once again to respond to life's stressors. The life force becomes more resilient and flexible. This manifests as overall physical, emotional, mental, and spiritual well-being. This state of balance translates into greater immunity and adaptability.

In constitutional treatment, homeopaths base their prescriptions on what they call the "totality of symptoms." This totality encompasses all discernable deviations from the normal healthy baseline. The underlying disturbance in the vital force can only be detected by its outward manifestations, by the symptoms it produces. This includes all physical, mental, and emotional symptoms as described by the patient. It was Hahnemann himself who first instructed his students to choose the *simillimum* by determining the totality of symptoms.

> *The totality of symptoms must be the principal or the only thing whereby the disease can make discernable what remedy it requires, the only thing that can determine the choice of the most suitable helping-means. Thus, in a word, the totality of symptoms must be the most important, indeed the only thing in every case of disease, that the medical-art practitioner has to discern and to clear away, by means of his art, so that the disease shall be cured and transformed into health.*[71]

This does not necessarily mean that a healthy person is one who is completely symptom free. The deciding factor is whether or not balance can be restored after symptoms appear. Think, for example, of normal immunologic milestones such as chicken pox or measles. Contrary to current medical thinking, these are not undesirable events. They are opportunities to hone the defensive skills of the immune system. By contracting and recovering successfully from illnesses of this nature, the immune system becomes stronger and more resilient. The life force is challenged, prevails, and grows and matures as a consequence.

On a more profound level, we can think of illness as both an impediment to and a catalyst for growth of consciousness. When the life force gets bogged down with chronic illness, it must expend additional energy compensating for and coping with its condition. That leaves less energy to deal with life's everyday demands. The consequence can be a slowing down of the maturation process. Psychological growth is harder to come by. Awareness is limited because extra effort is spent managing the pain and suffering that comes with illness. When chronic illness lasts for years it can serve as a significant roadblock to personal development.

On the other hand, the great paradox is that psychological growth is less likely to occur without a catalyst to encourage it. In this sense, suffering and illness are important factors that contribute to greater human consciousness. The critical determinant is how we manage to deal with the crosses that we must bear.

Medical therapies that combat symptoms have a distinct tendency to increase the likelihood that one will remain bogged down, stuck in place so to speak. Life's stressors are inevitable. Symptoms act as indicators that change and adaptability are required. When the life force successfully adapts, symptoms resolve and lessons are learned, regardless of whether we are fully conscious of those changes or not.

While pharmaceuticals can reduce pain and suffering in the short term, they often prevent the life force from restoring homeostasis. Suppression works at cross-purposes to the life force's natural inclinations and, in doing so, encourages chronicity of illness, thus making it more likely that growth of consciousness will be difficult to achieve.

Perhaps one of the greatest joys of being a homeopathic physician is having the privilege to witness the changes that take place as a consequence of a well-chosen homeopathic medicine. It is commonplace for patients to report back with personal epiphanies or revelatory dreams that teach them something profound regarding their struggles and the way in which those struggles contributed to their illnesses. Such insights are far from coincidental. They are a direct consequence of the freeing-up of the vital force.

In this sense, illness is nothing more than an indicator that there is a bioenergetic bottleneck, an obstruction to consciousness that needs tending to. Homeopathy does not just relieve pain and suffering. The dynamic action of a well-chosen homeopathic medicine can restore physical health and emotional balance, renew vitality, and promote greater awareness.

CHAPTER 9
Common Misconceptions

> *Homeopathy is not a philosophy, it is a principle.*
> –Margery Blackie, MD,
>   *Physician to Her Majesty, the Queen* (1976)
>
> *The history of homœopathy is the indictment of the medical profession.*
> –Wilhelm Ameke, MD (1883)

Homeopathy has been a continual target of derision since its inception in the time of Dr. Hahnemann. From day one it was viewed as a threat to the prevailing school of medical thought. And that same attitude continues to this day. Detractors have been known to spread a great deal of disinformation in attempts to discredit homeopathy. It is a truly challenging task to educate the public about homeopathy in the face of the misunderstandings created by so much false information.

With the rise of digital media, anti-homeopathy propaganda campaigns have become increasingly aggressive and sophisticated. Online efforts to undermine homeopathy are waged both overtly and covertly by organized groups of anti-holistic medicine militants who like to refer to themselves as "skeptics." There is widespread belief that PhRMA secretly funds some of these groups.

A skeptic's default position is that nothing can be considered credible unless science has already proven it to be true beyond a shadow of a doubt. Unlike real scientists who take a neutral stance on issues of scientific interest, skeptics begin from a position of disbelief. It is not hard to see how such an attitude would stifle all new and innovative ideas from the moment they are proposed. Think of it as the opposite of the *innocent until proven guilty* standard of the legal system.

Unfortunately, the medical profession has assimilated a good bit of this anti-homeopathy propaganda without stopping to question its sources. It is not uncommon to come across outspoken critics of homeopathy who literally know nothing about it besides the few talking points that they have absorbed from dishonest partisans.

I have written extensively about skepticism in *Metaphysics & Medicine*.[72] While skeptics see themselves as defenders of science, in actuality, they are promulgators of scientism. They are scientific fundamentalists who defend mainstream medicine as the one and only true source of medical knowledge. It is essential to be able to differentiate science from scientism, especially since the boundaries between the two have become increasingly blurred in contemporary culture.

Science was originally conceived as a systematic method of studying the world around us and within us. Eventually, it came to mean the study of the natural world, where *natural* meant the material world of physical objects. Over time it became co-opted by persons invested in an objectivist, reductionist, mechanist worldview. Subjectivity as defined by personal experience and human consciousness became taboo and unworthy of the efforts of real scientists. Anything other than the strictly material world was out of bounds as a subject of scientific scrutiny. Nature was thus severed from its connection to all subjective aspects of human experience. Modern science continues to work within the self-imposed limits of this framework.

Conventional medical science has been badly hampered by these same limitations ever since. As a result, it is unable to take into account the roles that emotion, thought, dreams, consciousness, bioenergetics and other factors play in health and illness without appearing to be unscientific. Of course, the original source of this built-in bias was the perceived need for medicine to distance itself from the superstitious thinking that it equated with religious doctrine. The irony is that modern medical science itself has become doctrinaire in the process. It has confined itself to a prison constructed from its own unacknowledged ideological beliefs.

Scientism is scientific ideology taken to an extreme. In its most elemental form, scientism is an exaggerated belief in the authority of science. Hardcore scientism asserts that scientific knowledge is the only real knowledge. Only science can provide access to truth. All other forms of human inquiry and experience are inferior and not to be trusted.

Skeptics frequently invoke the authority of science to make whatever claims they wish to make, regardless of the truth or accuracy of those claims. For example, in the name of science and without any evidence to back up their claims, skeptics are known to make statements like, "it is unscientific to question the safety of GMOs (genetically modified organisms)," or "vaccines do not cause harm." In similar fashion, they would lead people unfamiliar with the topic to believe that, "homeopathy is dangerous," or "homeopathy has been disproven."

Skeptics are the religious fanatics of the scientific world. While religious ideologues believe they speak with God's authority, skeptics mistakenly believe that they stand on the certainty of scientific authority. Skeptics wield their distorted scientistic beliefs as a weapon to discredit opposing beliefs that don't meet with their approval. Truth be told, skepticism is a malignancy that only serves to undermine legitimate science.

As defenders of conventional medical science, skeptics have taken it upon themselves to destroy homeopathy by any means possible, including subterfuge and dishonesty. The source of many misconceptions regarding homeopathy, therefore, can be traced back to skeptics' efforts to disseminate false information.

Here are just a few such distortions. Some have been perpetuated by skeptics, while others can be attributed to a simple lack of reliable information:

1. Homeopathic doses are too small to have any effect.
This is a false assertion that arises from the mistaken belief that all medicinal agents must act in a manner similar to conventional drugs. As we have seen, remedies are bioenergetic catalysts that are standardized by dilution factor and measured by the intensity and depth of effect they have on the people who take them. All homeopaths know that remedies do not act like drugs and, yet, critics insist that in order for homeopathic medicines to be taken seriously they must follow the principles of conventional pharmacology.

Skeptics refuse to acknowledge that remedies can have bioenergetic effects and, instead, continue to try to fit the round peg of homeopathic medicines into the square hole of pharmaceuticals. As with most criticisms of homeopathy, the claim that homeopathic doses are too small to work is based on theory, not experience. Since they do not work in accordance with conventional pharmaceutical standards—so the argument goes—they can't possibly work at all.

2. Homeopathy is not possible because it is implausible.
This is a remarkably closed-minded argument that assumes it is not possible for homeopathy to work because it makes no sense from a conventional medical perspective. Rather than opening one's mind to a different way of looking at things, the simple-minded skeptic, without further investigation, concludes that homeopathy doesn't work because it can't work.

This is the sort of nonsensical argument espoused by those who see themselves as defenders of science. It would be the equivalent of flat-earth theorists arguing that the earth can't be round because it contradicts the flat earth theory. Skeptics are famous for arguing that homeopathy defies the laws of chemistry and physics. This is a rather odd claim given the fact that there are a good number of contemporary scientists, including chemists and physicists, who are fascinated by homeopathy and are conducting research into its mechanism of action. Turning the tables, one can rightly claim that conventional medicine is flat earth medicine by virtue of the fact that it fails to acknowledge the roles that physics and energetics play in healing.

3. Homeopathy is pseudoscience.

This argument is a complete non-starter because, as far as I am concerned, there is no such thing as pseudoscience. It's just a snooty and obnoxious way of conveying the message that "your" science isn't real science because it's not like "our" science. Pseudoscience is just a word conjured up by those who feel the need to discredit ideas that threaten their beliefs. When you encounter the term, you know that you are dealing with a scientific ideologue. You might just as well substitute words like *heretic* or *idolater* and you'd get the same basic effect. Pseudoscience is a word that signifies intellectual intolerance on the part of the person using it.

Notwithstanding the silliness of the pseudoscience argument, homeopathic methodology is about as close to true classical science as one can get. Substances are studied in a non-biased way via provings in order to determine their symptom profiles. The symptom pattern of the patient is matched with a substance that is capable of causing symptoms similar to that pattern. The matching substance is administered in homeopathic dosage, the response is observed, and the results are recorded. Homeopathic methodology epitomizes the very definition of systematic empirical observation and experiment.

4. There is no scientific evidence to support homeopathy.

This is perhaps the most commonly repeated lie about homeopathy. Although it is a flat out falsehood, skeptics have made the claim so often that it has become a virtual internet meme. Notwithstanding, there are literally thousands of research trials involving homeopathy.

One particular review concluded that the percentage of homeopathic studies that yield positive results (41%)[73] is quite similar to the percentage of orthodox medical trials that yield positive results (44%).[74] These numbers are remarkable given that conventional research protocols are not particularly compatible with the manner in which homeopathy is practiced. In order to satisfy conventional research protocols, the key component of homeopathic practice—individualized treatment—must often be sacrificed in the name of allopathic standardization and homogeneity. It's like trying to evaluate quantum physics according to the standards of classical Newtonian physics; it's just not possible

Nevertheless, even when homeopathy is squeezed into an allopathic mold of evaluation, the results are just as good as studies of conventional medicine. One has to wonder what the results would reveal if research methods were more appropriately adjusted to homeopathic standards of practice.

5. Homeopathy is dangerous.

The claim here is that patients who need "real" medicine will not receive it and will be harmed if they waste their time with homeopathic care. This is a rather desperate argument that fails to account for the fact that all practitioners and healers are held to the same basic standard. All, including homeopaths, conventional doctors, and unconventional doctors, must acknowledge their limitations and make appropriate referrals when necessary.

This argument makes one big whopper of an assumption, which is that conventional medicine has all the answers to all problems at all times. In other words, when you fail to partake of all that conventional medicine has to offer, you place yourself in grave danger. It is possible to completely reverse this argument by noting that, given the remarkably high rates of morbidity and mortality associated with conventional medical treatment, it is wise to seek alternative care before subjecting oneself to allopathic danger. Of course, I don't believe this either. Every situation is unique. Some are ideal for homeopathic treatment; others are better suited for allopathic care. It all depends on the circumstances.

6. Homeopathy may benefit people psychologically, but it can't treat real organic disease.

Skeptics admit that there can be psychological benefits from homeopathic care but then explain it away as a function of the attention given by homeopathic practitioners to their patients. I don't doubt that the time I spend with my patients has its positive benefits. I also know that no simple talk therapy, or extended psychotherapy for that matter, can yield the kinds of results that millions of homeopathic consumers have experienced firsthand.

Often within weeks of beginning homeopathic treatment patients have been known to report significant progress with issues that they have struggled with for years. For example, feelings of lack of confidence can diminish rapidly, thus altering the course of a person's life. Persons who have struggled for years with symptoms related to PTSD may report greater calm and less inclination toward aggression. Children terrified of the dark are suddenly able to sleep alone at night, thus relieving parents of their worry and stress. These are routine stories that all good homeopaths can recount from their clinical experiences.

The same types of outcomes apply to homeopathic treatment of physical health conditions, both functional and organic. I use homeopathy on a regular basis to successfully treat conditions like bronchitis, pneumonia, bladder infections, skin rashes, warts, ovarian cysts, colitis, constipation, arthritis, and much more. The notion that homeopathy is not effective for organic pathology is just a biased extension of the idea that homeopathy doesn't work because it can't work. In other words, that argument doesn't have a leg to stand on.

Of course, none of the above claims would ordinarily require a dignified response. Since skeptics use deceit, dishonesty, and disingenuous tactics to purposefully undermine homeopathy, there is no obligation to provide answers to their objections or treat their phony claims with respect. Unfortunately, their disinformation campaigns do have an impact on public opinion and, therefore, need to be rebutted. I also believe that the best defense is a good offense. Singing the praises of the miracle of homeopathy is a far better strategy than bickering with willfully pigheaded naysayers.

7. If homeopathy is legitimate, it must meet the standards of "this for that" treatment.

This is the idea that all medicinal agents must have specific purposes. In other words, they must be designed to target specific symptoms. You know what I mean—Pepcid is for heartburn, Zyrtec is for allergies, Xanax is for anxiety, and so on. This is not so much a skeptic talking point as much as a general belief engendered by our conventionally oriented medical culture. We simply assume that all drugs work in a "this drug for that condition" manner.

This is why so many of us wind up taking multiple drugs for our various symptomatic complaints. This is often compounded by the fact that we take additional drugs for the new problems created by the initial drugs.

Given this prevailing mindset, it is near impossible to grasp the basic premise of homeopathy, which is so fundamentally different from mainstream society's standards of medical care. It makes no sense whatsoever to say that *Pulsatilla* is for ear infections. While *Pulsatilla* can help ear infections, it has also been known to treat diarrhea, coughs, arthritis, grief, unassertiveness, and much more. All remedies have multiple indications, far too many to fit on any label.

The true purpose of any homeopathic prescription is to treat the whole person. It is not intended to treat the illness, per se, as much as the person with the illness. Breaking through that conventional medical programming and reeducating patients about the nature of homeopathic healing can be a time consuming process.

To make matters worse, homeopathic medicines usually come in pill form, thus perpetuating the notion that each remedy must have a specific indication. In the U.S., the FDA (Food and Drug Administration) does nothing to dispel this idea. It legally requires that the labels of homeopathic medicines list what condition or symptoms they are intended to treat. One has to wonder whether this is indicative of how poorly FDA understands homeopathy or whether it represents a deliberate attempt to undermine homeopathy by forcing it to conform to conventional medical standards.

8. Homeopathy is not a science. It is a philosophical belief system.

There are some who argue that homeopathy is not a science. It is just a fanciful, made-up, New Age philosophy, they say. And the reader might ask, haven't I been writing about that homeopathic philosophy in this book? Yes, I have, but that doesn't mean homeopathy is a philosophy. The philosophy I write about is a by-product of the lessons learned from the day-to-day practice of homeopathic principles.

Homeopathy is based upon a principle—the principle of similars—around which is built a methodology, the results of which make one reflect back upon the nature of health and illness. Hahnemann first observed the principle of similars in action when he studied the effects of Peruvian bark. He then devised a methodology to test that principle to see if it applied to more than just the one example. From this he constructed a system of healing called homeopathy. All discussions in this book about the nature of disease, the role of the psyche in illness, the direction of cure, the bioenergetic nature of homeopathic dilutions, and so on, are conclusions drawn from having repeatedly observed homeopathy in action. The empirical experience gained from homeopathic practice precedes homeopathic theory and philosophy.

Now let's compare this to conventional medicine, which proudly calls itself the "rational" medicine. Orthodox medicine constructs all manner of scientific theories, which it then seeks to superimpose upon nature. For example, germs are theorized to be the cause of many illnesses. Drugs that can kill those bugs are manufactured and administered. Germ theory has its advantages but it also has its limitations. The war on germs has now reached its historical denouement and the fallout isn't looking pretty.

Medicine turns a blind eye to the flaws inherent in germ theory. It chooses instead to forge ahead, insisting that its worldview is correct despite the protestations of nature. The same strategy that failed to conquer bacterial disease is now being pursued in the war against viral illness. It doesn't take a genius to realize that we will someday have to contend with the scourge of drug-resistant super-viruses.

Biotechnology and genetic engineering are also consequences of man-made medical theories imposed upon nature. I believe that the unforeseen repercussions of unchecked biotech will far outweigh the benefits. The fallout will be grave indeed. This illustrates the dangers that can arise when orthodox medicine is misguidedly beholden to its pet theories. The great edifice of scientific medicine has been constructed not around empirical fact, but around a set of highly dubious theoretical beliefs—like the belief that an unyielding war against microbes is a winning strategy. Medicine arrogantly demands that human illness conform to its philosophy.

Homeopathic theory is formulated after the fact, by virtue of the lessons learned from clinical experience. Orthodox medicine has it backwards. It constructs rational theories about human illness beforehand, and then seeks to confirm those theories afterwards in the clinic. Facts that do not support the latest theory are often ignored for the sake of preserving theory. Medicine, therefore, is a truly *rational* system of medical thought in the sense that it ignores empirical facts in the pursuit of its mentally constructed *theoretical* imperatives. While homeopathy is experience-based, allopathy is thought-based. In this sense, conventional medicine is much more akin to a philosophical belief system than is homeopathy.

9. Homeopathic medicines are nothing more than placebos.
While scientists have a tendency to make the placebo effect debate sound rather complex, it's really quite simple. In essence, the placebo effect boils down to the power of the mindbody to heal itself. Anything that supports a person's efforts to heal also tends to enhance the placebo effect. Although it is a ubiquitous phenomenon, the placebo effect is not necessarily distributed evenly throughout all healing modalities.

A case can be made for the idea that placebo effects are greater in more elaborate settings like large hospitals with expensive equipment and armies of personnel dressed in uniforms. It is also reasonable to think that placebo effects will be greater for culturally accepted medical therapies that have public support behind them. Again, we'll put the check mark here in orthodox medicine's column. An unprecedented amount of manpower, faith, and scientific effort has gone into the construction of the medical-industrial complex. How could it not have an enormous placebo effect on those who believe in it—and sometimes even those who do not?

For critics to claim that little old universally maligned homeopathy works only by virtue of the placebo effect is a rather ridiculous assertion. I can make a pretty good case for the opposite argument, which is that all the negative attention tends to work against homeopathy. It is not uncommon for a female patient who has experienced the benefits of homeopathy to urge her husband to also seek treatment. When the husband begins his consultation by warning me that he is only there at the urging of his wife and that he is skeptical of homeopathy, the net effect is to diminish any potential placebo effect.

When critics argue that the extended time spent with patients and the attention paid to detail by homeopathic practitioners is conducive of a placebo effect, I do not dispute that. It's quite common for homeopathic patients to remark that they have never had a doctor take their concerns so seriously. Such comments should be read as a not so flattering commentary on the impersonal nature of conventional medical care. Charges that homeopathic medicines are placebos amounts to a classic case of the pot calling the kettle black. There is no greater placebo effect than that which accompanies mainstream medicine.

The placebo effect is everywhere, whether we are willing to admit it or not. In the final analysis, it boils down to a question of whether the effects produced by homeopathy are exclusively placebo effects or whether there is more to it. Does homeopathy work above and beyond placebo? The answer, of course, is a resounding yes!

On a daily basis, I make it my business to determine whether the outcomes reported by my patients are comparatively short-lived and superficial, which is to be expected in the case of most placebo responses, or whether the effects are more global and long lasting as one would expect from an accurate homeopathic prescription. While the placebo effect does represent a version of the body's attempt to heal itself it, unfortunately, commonly falls short of the mark—which is why it needs a nudge in the right direction from a bioenergetic stimulus that can enhance that effect. Homeopathy does just that.

Meanwhile, instead of seeking to maximize the self-healing power of the mindbody, conventional medicine looks at the placebo effect as an annoyance that gets in the way of its pursuit of "real" medicine. Clinical research trials, for example, seek to isolate and account for placebo effects so that they do not pollute their findings. The bottom line is that specious arguments that homeopathy is nothing more than placebo medicine almost always come from those with a premeditated bias against it.

Paradigm wars

Of course, all the fuss makes one wonder why there is so much animosity toward homeopathy. Shouldn't healers of all stripes, conventional and otherwise, be thrilled to hear about innovative methods that can benefit their patients? One might think so, but this is often not the case. Instead, we tend to see knee-jerk challenges to newly proposed ideas, even before they have had a fair hearing.

Patients who have experienced the benefits of homeopathy are often puzzled over why there would be so much resistance from the medical profession to something that works so well. Sad to say, while we tend to put physicians on a pedestal, they are people just like the rest of us. Even men and women of science are subject to personal biases that can cloud their vision and blind them to new healing truths.

With that said, there must be more to mainstream resistance than human nature—and I believe that there is. The concept of scientific paradigms and paradigm shifts is widely attributed to Thomas S. Kuhn, an American philosopher of science.[75] He defined the practice of "normal science" as science conducted within the parameters of the prevailing scientific paradigm. It is conducted without questioning the underlying assumptions of what is believed to be the settled science of the time. Most doctors and medical scientists practice normal science. They do not question the basic foundational paradigmatic beliefs of Western medicine. Medical education, regulation, and professionalization serve to ensure that physicians do not question the fundamental assumptions of the mainstream medical paradigm.

Homeopathy operates outside the bounds of the conventional medical paradigm. Which is to say that homeopathic medicine and orthodox medicine have two completely different perspectives regarding the nature of health, illness, and healing. They function within different paradigms and operate by different sets of rules. Their foundational beliefs diverge so widely as to make it difficult to find common ground. There is a tendency to talk past each other as if the two are speaking different languages. Fortunately, many homeopathic practitioners also have conventional medical training, which, to some extent, serves to bridge the gap. Although most orthodox physicians have little knowledge of the subject, it doesn't seem to deter some from expressing their strong opposition to homeopathy.

Professor Kuhn wrote about the idea of scientific anomalies, which are pieces of information that don't quite fit into the conceptual framework of the prevailing paradigm. They tend to be pushed aside so that the business of normal science can continue. However, when the number of anomalies reaches critical mass, when they can no longer be ignored, a change in scientific paradigms becomes possible. I believe that we are fast approaching that point with Western medical science.

Across the board we are witnessing all sorts of mini-crises within the medical profession. There are so many that it is no longer possible to ignore them. Drug-resistant bacteria, growing lists of shocking side effects openly acknowledged in television commercials, dangerous drugs pulled off the market, out-of-control medical expenses, institutional corruption, old research findings overturned by new research findings—the list of glaring problems goes on. Many of these events constitute anomalies that have arisen because of or in spite of the practice of normal medical science. The solution to these problems requires an ability to step outside of the mainstream medical paradigm in order to consider them from a new perspective. That new perspective is the holistic paradigm within which homeopathic medicine thrives.

Old ideas don't often die easily. Failing to understand that its lack of conceptual framework is the source of its problems, medicine chooses instead to defend its ideas to the bitter end, and that means fighting to maintain control and doing battle against the very ideas that could help solve its problems. Resistance to change is compounded by the sad reality that so much money continues to be made through the practice of bad medicine.

We live in a world in which most people are aligned with conventional medicine. They have assimilated a certain way of thinking about health and illness that has led to a variety of dead ends, the repercussions of which are becoming increasingly clear. A growing number of dissatisfied medical consumers and alternative health practitioners are aware of these problems. They have made it their mission to seek new methods of healing. In their search for answers, many have come to realize that the overall conceptual framework needs to change. It's not just a matter of continuing to search for solutions within the existing framework of normal medical science. The framework itself must change. The time has come for a quantum leap in perspective. A paradigm shift is in order.

The current state of cultural polarization sweeping the globe is an additional factor serving to exacerbate the medical and scientific paradigm wars. The false dichotomy working its way into mainstream consciousness is that you are either pro-science or anti-science. Pro-science people are well educated, intelligent, and rational, while those who question corporate science are ignorant, crazy people who make decisions based on emotion. The source of this phony rhetoric of division can be traced to those with an economic stake in maintaining the status quo.

Of course, the idea that there is no middle ground is ridiculous. The ascent of the new holistic paradigm does not have to mean the annihilation of the old school paradigm. Modern medicine has made many positive contributions to healthcare. But it also seems to have run out of good ideas. The rise of biotechnology has little to do with real healing and everything to do with the exploitation of markets. The number of casualties resulting from this ruthless trend can only be expected to rise.

The pitfalls and dangers of mainstream medicine have become impossible to ignore. It is time that we acknowledge those problems and make room for new ideas. It is time to reevaluate orthodox medicine's failing war against disease. Holistic methods of treatment take a more cooperative approach to healing. They seek to work with the life force rather than fight against it. Both medical paradigms have their advantages and their shortcomings. It is possible to incorporate the best of both into a system that works for the benefit of all.

Theory and experience

There are enough differences between conventional and homeopathic medicine to warrant their placement in different medical paradigms. Although those differences are many, there is one particular factor that I believe deserves special attention. It is a difference that divides the two at the level of their core foundational beliefs. The same factor goes to the very heart of the culture and science wars, which are increasingly threatening to divide society into polarized camps.

Contrary to the popular belief that the problem lies with scientifically illiterate persons who are not capable of making judgments regarding new scientific developments, I believe that the real source of the widening divide is science's growing tendency to overstep the bounds of its authority. Scientific opinion is gradually filling the vacuum left behind by religion's fading dominance. We are increasingly expected to believe the pronouncements of science regardless of the thinness of supporting evidence and in spite of the fickle nature of scientific opinion, which seems to shift with each new research study.

The general public is justifiably skeptical of a scientific establishment that has assimilated the characteristics of the religious institutional authorities that it has displaced. The historical struggle between religion and science is a function of their mutual imperialistic impulses. Both have a tendency to become autocratic when given too much power.

There is no doubt that scientific experts should be the ones to conduct new research and implement new technologies. However, there is no justification to exclude others from the decision-making process. Both government and the general public are adequately qualified to determine whether they wish to support or reject the initiatives proposed by the scientific establishment. They rightly serve as a system of checks and balances so that science does not get carte blanche to do whatever it chooses.

Given the chance, mainstream medicine would move to eliminate the competition represented by alternative forms of health and healing. However, the general public clearly thinks otherwise. They overwhelmingly prefer to have options and do not wish to have public policy dictated to them by those who control the delivery of medical services. The average person prefers choice for a number of non-scientific reasons, the most important of which has to do with personal experience. The public forms its opinions based on information gathered from family, friends, news sources, and more. They don't ignore the science; they just believe that science is not the be-all and end-all when it comes to the decision-making process.

Science has so thoroughly dissociated its activities from the human factor that it often cannot see itself the way others do. Its devastating impact upon human and environmental health is increasingly apparent to many. How has this come to be? Why is modern science so oblivious of and insensitive to human considerations? The answer has to do with its allegiance to rationality.

Science is a victim of its own methodology, its exceedingly rational way of approaching problems. Science strictly limits itself to the information provided by logic and reason. Now at first blush, that doesn't sound so bad. Isn't science supposed to be objective and dispassionate? Well, yes—and no. Objectivity is important but science has taken it to such an extreme that it now defines subjectivity as untrustworthy and irrelevant. Through a seriously flawed leap of logic scientists have eggheadedly convinced themselves that since personal experience is subjective, it can no longer be considered a valid form of evidence.

In medicine, this translates into the idea that patients' direct feedback to their doctors is far less important than the data provided by the scientific literature. Science uses "anecdotal evidence" as a dismissive term to emphasize the unreliability of patient experience. Reading between the lines, "anecdotal" conveys the message that laypersons don't know any better and should, therefore, let the scientists do all the serious thinking. To denigrate patient experience in such a manner is not scientific; it's a gross demonstration of bias.

Modern science has erected a wall of denial when it comes to human experience. It is slave to its own rationally constructed theories. It trusts its own logic more than the wisdom that comes from experience. Because it is so ferociously beholden to its rationalizations, and because it disregards the feedback provided by the people it is supposed to serve, science cannot always be trusted to do the right thing.

In medicine, that means pursuing the war against microbes to the bitter end, regardless of the long-term consequences. It means the continued production of an endless string of vaccines regardless of growing evidence that they are implicated in a broad spectrum of problems including previously unheard of autoimmune diseases. It means that GMOs (genetically modified organisms) inserted into the food chain are presumed to be harmless until proven otherwise—in spite of the protestations of concerned citizens.

At the heart of the culture wars is one very important unaccounted-for factor. As a civilization, we are evolving away from unquestioning obedience to external forms of authority and toward greater reliance upon personal experience as a guide. Many are beginning to question scientific authority, especially when it comes to personal health decisions. Add to this a growing suspicion of corporate sponsored science and you have the conditions ripe for a paradigmatic revolution.

Enter homeopathy, which meets with tremendous resistance from mainstream medicine because it takes issue with conventional concepts of health, illness, and healing. Homeopathy is an almost exclusively empirical medical therapy. It is a practical, hands-on methodology that relies on patient experience as its primary source of information—the very same information that orthodoxy dismisses as unreliably anecdotal.

The clash of worldviews is readily apparent. Skeptics say that homeopathy can't work because the doses are too small. Homeopaths respond that homeopathic medicines do not act through biochemical means. They act as bioenergetic catalysts. Skeptics counter that that is impossible; it defies what we know of chemistry and physics. Homeopaths question, then how do you account for the fact that my patients keep getting better? Skeptics answer that that's just anecdotal evidence. There is no scientific proof that homeopathy works. Homeopaths reply that they prefer to trust their firsthand clinical experiences regardless of what the conventional scientific literature says (and notwithstanding the fact that there is plenty of research to support the beneficial effects of homeopathy). As long as our patients get better, that is all that counts.

And round and round the argument goes. The contentious debate clearly illustrates the primary difference between the two medical paradigms. One side trusts the logic of their rationally constructed theories about the nature of illness while the other trusts their clinical experiences and the experiences of their patients. One is fundamentally rational while the other is empirical. One side emphasizes theory while the other relies on experience.

The same debate is indicative of a larger cultural divide between mainstream rational thought and alternative holistic ways of approaching societal problems. We think so much that we have lost touch with ourselves, with our emotions, our intuition, our values, and our capacity to integrate all those faculties, including the rational faculty, into a well-rounded whole. Correspondingly, patients have lost touch with personal experience and instead tend to think about their illnesses in purely abstract terms.

This is why, for example, when I ask a patient to tell me about his arthritis he says something like the following. "My doctor says it's rheumatoid arthritis. It is an autoimmune condition that causes inflammation of my joints. I have an elevated sed rate and a positive rheumatoid factor. My anti-inflammatory medication helps some but not enough. I don't want to take the stronger medication that my doctor is recommending." Clearly, this patient is well versed in mainstream medical thinking. Unfortunately, he has told me nothing homeopathically useful about his problem. Instead, he has provided a synopsis of conventional medical theory regarding arthritis and its diagnosis.

Now contrast this with the type of answer that I am looking for when I ask about a person's arthritis. "It began five years ago after the death of my father. My marriage was also under a great deal of strain at the time. I thought I was going to lose my wife. The pain and swelling began in both knees. The pain eventually spread to both shoulders. It's an aching sensation that seems to get worse around 9 or 10 in the morning. It's also worse in hot weather. I swear that it acts up when I'm under emotional stress. Since this all began, I've also developed a tendency to get a lot of mouth sores." (Remedy choice?[76])

Let's try a third example of a person who has been told she has arthritis. "I feel stiffness and pain in my joints, especially my left knee and left shoulder. It's hard to get going in the morning because I'm so stiff, but once I get moving around it's not as bad. My chiropractor gave my some stretching exercises to do, which seem to help. Cold rainy weather really bothers it a lot. If I sit for too long I have more trouble. As long as I keep moving or take a hot shower I manage to survive." (Remedy choice?[77])

Examples two and three are descriptions of firsthand experience. Note that the two descriptions are quite different. It would be hard to mistake one for the other. The second example has a strong psychological component. The third seems more physical. Compare these two examples to the first case, which tells us literally nothing about that individual's experience of arthritis. The information provided in the first case would be sufficient for any conventional doctor to initiate drug therapy. A homeopathic doctor would need much more information before being able to decide on a plan of action.

Note that the first example is a cookie-cutter theory-based explanation that could apply to most if not all cases of rheumatoid arthritis. It is an explanation of the theoretical cause and/or mechanism behind rheumatoid arthritis. It is not a description of symptomatic experience. Allopathic theories regarding disease causation tend to change over time. As the theories change so do the therapies.

The second and third examples are experience-based empirical descriptions that will always remain the same. Since homeopathic treatment depends on experience and not theory, patient number three will benefit from the same remedy as another patient who describes a similar symptom pattern fifty years from now. The homeopathic treatment will remain unchanged regardless of the allopathic theory of the day.

Homeopathy is phenomenological in nature. It takes patient experience at face value. It does not pass judgment. It does not question its truth or search for scientific explanations as to why patients have certain symptomatic experiences. When a person with depression reports that he has a tendency to blame himself for others' problems, the homeopath accepts that as the patient's experiential truth, and does not try to convince the patient of the falseness of his feelings. Neither does homeopathy propose theories involving neurotransmitters in order to be able to explain the reason for the patient's depression.

No, the homeopath takes the patient's report seriously and inquires further in order to get an accurate description of the symptom. If he reports that his self-blame is related to an inability to assert himself, the homeopath considers certain remedies known to fit that symptom. If the self-blame comes from a general feeling of unworthiness, the homeopath considers other remedies. The objective reality of the symptom or ability to explain its existence in medical terms is irrelevant. Descriptive accuracy is what matters most.

Conventional medicine proudly claims to be rational, which is true, but it also claims to be highly empirical, which is clearly not true. And therein lies the crux of the matter. Medicine has lost touch with its empirical roots. It has forgotten what true empiricism is all about. The irony is that it considers homeopathy unscientific because it relies on empirical experience and questions the logic of mainstream beliefs. The bottom line is that orthodox medicine consistently overlooks the importance of patient experience. Rational medicine downplays the value of physician's firsthand experiences and the experiences of their patients.

I can't honestly say that we are entering an age of rebirth, one that will restore experiential authority to its proper place—but it is sorely needed. The ability to trust one's own judgment and intuition is strongly conditioned by one's experiences. Our rational age of rational science and rational medicine has spawned generations of people who no longer feel that their own experiences carry any weight in a science-dominated culture.

In the final analysis, the lack of satisfactory scientific explanation for homeopathy doesn't mean a whit. All that matters is that homeopathy works, whether skeptics are willing to believe it or not. The answer to our modern day dilemma is a return to balance, to an approach to life's problems that values both rational thought and experiential truth. Homeopathy provides an experienced-based model for healing that does not depend upon being able to explain everything in scientific terms. It offers a beacon of hope for a thought-based culture that has lost touch with the very thing that makes us all human, the truth and validity of our personal experiences.

CHAPTER 10

The Revolutionary Nature of Homeopathic Healing

> *The animal kingdom has in itself the image of sickness, and the vegetable and mineral kingdoms in like manner, and if man were perfectly conversant with the substances of these three kingdoms he could treat the whole human race.*
>
> –James Tyler Kent, MD (1919)

> *The emergence of homeopathic medicine ... represents a revolution of thought in its approach to illness. Not only did its theories, practice and methods propose a radical change from the medicine being practised in Hahnemann's lifetime but they still represent a view of reality somewhat at loggerheads with contemporary scientific and medical beliefs.*
>
> –Elizabeth Danciger (1987)

Orthodox medicine from a homeopathic perspective

All my years of hearing patients' stories about their encounters with the medical system gives me a unique perspective, one that allows me to compare homeopathic to conventional treatment. Knowing what I now know, orthodox medicine really is quite simplistic by comparison. Don't get me wrong. Medicine has much to offer, but it also has some significant shortcomings.

How are we to know what changes are in order if we can't honestly and openly critique medicine's flaws? Likewise, how are people to know that viable alternatives exist if they are not given adequate and accurate information? That is my purpose here, to highlight the pluses and minuses so that people are aware of their options.

Perhaps the most glaring issue is that medicine is committed to a therapeutic strategy that guarantees a never-ending pipeline of new and often toxic drugs. It is not possible to anticipate the impact of new synthetic substances that have never before existed. The full range of potential direct effects, side effects, and long-term effects of a drug cannot be truly known before it is brought to market. As a result, the dangers are acknowledged far too late, only after a drug has taken its toll.

It is near impossible to anticipate how drugs will affect the health of the ecosystem. The harmful relationship between pharmaceuticals and the environment is very difficult and expensive to prove. The degree of difficulty creates a perfect opportunity for continued malfeasance and denial of culpability on the part of companies that manufacture these drugs.

I have a hard time understanding how a medical system can be so invested in the belief that manmade synthetic chemicals would provide the best answers to human illness. It is a testament to the closed nature of modern medical education, which seems virtually impervious to new ideas. Corporate influence, shrewd marketing, professional indoctrination, and science conducted by vested interests constitute a powerful and toxic mix.

Mainstream medicine's shortsighted thinking is another problematic issue. A medical philosophy that thinks no further than the elimination of the most immediate symptoms is a recipe for serious trouble. The sad truth is that medicine is not even conscious of the suppressive nature of the drugs it employs. As long as it remains unaware, it does not have to acknowledge the longer-term consequences of its actions. It does what it does without pangs of conscience.

Furthermore, suppression creates a vicious cycle of consumers who will always be in need of more medical services. Rather than examine the root causes of this revolving door of medical need, the medical system looks the other way, content to be the beneficiary of short-term solutions that engender long-term problems.

Another stubborn problem is medicine's inability to acknowledge the reality of the mindbody unity. Medicine gives lip service to the concept of psychological stress while denying the proper place of mind in the etiology of illness. If, as I would contend, most illness has its roots in psychological/emotional disturbances, then why does medicine continue to promote only physiological/biological solutions? The answer, of course, is that medicine is mired in a materialist philosophy. Even though many doctors would privately acknowledge the role of mind and emotion in the development of disease, to speak of the idea openly in a professional setting would be to subject oneself to accusations of being unscientific.

Science is concerned only with the concrete. It has no interest in something as elusive and intangible as human consciousness because its limited worldview does not account for it. Stress, therefore, is really just a convenient dumping ground for all sorts of phenomena that medical science feels inadequate to handle. Consciousness is ubiquitous, but because it cannot be seen, touched, or quantified, the scientific mind has no idea what to do with it.

A medical therapy that cannot account for consciousness will always fall short of true healing. If mind and body are one, then focusing only on the physical manifestations of illness will yield superficial results. Splitting mindbody into two, with one to be treated by the doctor and the other by the psychotherapist, will also produce unsatisfactory results. By contrast, homeopathy acknowledges the reality of the mindbody unity and has a practical means to treat it as the one single entity that it is.

One consequence of this lack of understanding of the mindbody is an overemphasis on will power. When medicine fails, patients are told to tough it out and to reduce their stress levels. In other words, they are led to believe that if they just try hard enough they can will themselves to wellness. It amounts to another subtle form of blame. The net effect is to make patients feel bad about themselves when they are unable to overcome their illnesses.

This uniquely American brand of rugged individualism is both immature and counterproductive. It shames people into downplaying or ignoring their psychological suffering. This applies especially to men who are nurtured on the cultural myth that they must be able to persevere through all manner of emotional difficulties without help and without complaining. How often have you heard someone say, "Don't cry?" The message is deeply ingrained in the American psyche and medicine does little to dispel such illness-engendering attitudes.

Homeopathy doesn't shove psychological symptoms aside in order to get to the "real" physical problems. Most people's problems are neither physical nor psychological. They are, in actuality, energetic disturbances that know no boundaries and can, therefore, manifest in any number of ways. A man's tendency toward irritability requires just as much attention as his chronic back pain. A woman's anxiety over the safety of her children is just as important as her irritable bowel symptoms. When homeopathic treatment works, the patient begins to feel better both in mind and body.

Another problem is medicine's overemphasis on diagnostics. When treatment fails, the default mode is to run more diagnostics. When a mindbody problem doesn't respond to physical intervention, medicine assumes the failure is due to diagnostic error. Specialists are consulted and more tests are conducted in the hope that if a correct diagnosis can be made the problem can be solved. Sometimes this is a worthwhile pursuit but, more often than not, it subjects patients to unnecessary testing that can be invasive and risky. It is my belief that this overemphasis on testing is really just a form of diagnostic distraction. Running more tests allows everyone involved to believe that the situation is under control and a solution may be imminent.

A related problem discussed earlier is diagnostic stereotyping. Prefabricated diagnostic categories do a disservice to real patients whose ailments often do not conform to those categories. Instead of responding appropriately to treatment failure by modifying its faulty perspective, medicine persists in imposing its artificial disease taxonomy upon patients in the name of efficiency and one-size-fits-all treatment. The result is far from efficient and less than satisfactory.

For example, debating whether or not a child has attention deficit disorder (ADD) is not a critical part of the homeopathic evaluation process. It's neither here nor there. It's just a label, which would be meaningless if it did not carry such a societal stigma. It might be meaningful if orthodox medicine had effective treatment for it, but it does not—unless one is willing to have one's child take pharmaceutical grade amphetamines on an indefinite basis.

Since conventional medicine has little to offer such children, it busies itself instead with diagnostic debates that give one the impression of serious scientific import but which really don't amount to a hill of beans. Homeopaths understand that each child who carries the ADD label is unique. The individual details of each case—not the diagnostic label—help to determine the correct homeopathic prescription.

Some parents don't want their child to be given the ADD label because they are dead set against drug therapy. Others actively seek out the diagnosis in the hope that treatment will bring relief. Some look the other way, having convinced themselves that "kids will be kids," or that their children will eventually "grow out of it." Debating whether ADD—or chronic fatigue or irritable bowel syndrome or chronic Lyme disease for that matter—is a real thing is both a waste of time and an insult to patients who struggle with such problems. It is an artificial issue created by a medical system that stereotypes illness in ways that do not do justice to the diversity of human illness and the holistic reality of each individual suffering person.

On a deeper level, modern medicine has lost sight of the fundamentals of scientific method. Orthodox medicine is more rational than it is empirical. It favors a certain logic regarding the nature of illness and its treatment. It is reluctant to amend various theories that spring from this logic in spite of mounting empirical evidence indicating that those theories are flawed. Sound scientific method does not construct a logical proposition and then proceed to do whatever it takes to manufacture supporting evidence to prove that proposition, especially when such proof entails highly questionable statistical trickery and an ability to turn a blind eye to conflicting evidence. If it takes so much effort to justify a theory or therapy, then one has to question its validity. Shouldn't the most reliable indication of the value of a therapy be whether it helps patients get better and stay better without inordinate risk?

While conventional medicine gives the impression that it is a highly rigorous scientific enterprise, I believe that many of its problems stem from having deviated from true scientific method in the pursuit of validating its pet theories. Rational medicine is an elaborately constructed network of self-fulfilling logical propositions that, upon closer examination, turns out to be a rather irrational deviation from true empirical science.

But there is a larger issue here, and that is the fact that orthodox medicine inappropriately seeks to impose its rationally constructed theories upon the holistic reality of its patients. Its beliefs, practices, and imperialistic impulses inevitably come into conflict with the personal experiences of sick people. The net effect is to invalidate patient experience, all in the name of staying true to its unholistic beliefs. The inescapable result is a growing number of dissatisfied patients who have found that mainstream medicine's worldview clashes with their own.

Put plainly, many sick people seek conventional medical care, are given diagnoses that seem to make logical sense, are told that a particular treatment is the best option available, and that holistic therapies are just scams, only to find out after all is said and done that the treatment didn't work, or even worse, that the treatment left them sicker than when they first sought care. Cookie-cutter medicine doesn't always produce the best results.

Patients are left with two options. One is to override their perceptions regarding the nature of their own ailments. They quickly learn that their own personal observations are not particularly relevant to the medical system. As a consequence, they begin to disregard their firsthand experiences. Instead, they replace those experiences with a scientific language that reflects a vague and generalized stereotype of their actual problems. They slowly but surely learn to assimilate the conventional medical worldview and its attendant jargon as their own.

The second option is a daunting one, one that can require courage and fortitude. And that is to question the fundamental premises of orthodox medicine. The cognitive dissonance created by patients' encounters with the medical system cause many to search for answers that can only be found outside the bounds of the conventional medical paradigm. More and more are successfully navigating this uncharted territory and have discovered alternative approaches to meet their needs.

The death and rebirth of experience

One of the tragic side effects of our scientific age of rational thought is that we are losing touch with our inner selves. We are constantly reminded that our feelings, intuitive hunches, and even our values don't mean much. Only the so-called facts matter. Science doesn't care about what you think or feel. It's the data that counts. The scary truth is that we have collectively swallowed this unhealthy message. We have fallen for the big lie that science knows better than we do, particularly when it comes to matters of our own health.

Consider the fact that if you dare to challenge the medical system you may find yourself in legal trouble. I recall having to submit to an interrogation from a school superintendent after my attorney sent the district a letter notifying them that I refused on religious grounds to vaccinate my child. The superintendent openly admitted to me that he was very uncomfortable about having been placed in the position of having to judge the authenticity of my religious beliefs. If I failed the test, I would be forced to have my child vaccinated. The experts apparently knew more about what was best for my child than I did, notwithstanding the fact that I have a medical degree. The good news is that the superintendent was sympathetic to my situation.

We have unwittingly assimilated the message that qualitative experience-based knowledge is far less valuable than science-based quantitative knowledge. The primary consequence of having adopted this belief is that our capacity for self-knowledge has atrophied from neglect. Our capacity for critical judgment has also suffered. We no longer know how we really feel or what it is that we truly believe.

While patients struggle to describe the experiential nature of their health issues, they have no problem at all reciting medical doctrine regarding those illnesses. A patient tells me that his leg pain is due to nerve impingement at the fifth lumber vertebrae, but is at a loss for words when I ask him to describe what type of pain it is. Another patient tells me that she is tired because she is not getting enough REM sleep, but can't recall the dramatic dream she had two nights ago because she didn't think it was important enough to commit to memory. It has become far too easy to rationalize away our feelings and experiences.

A doctor can't describe the intimate details of a particular patient's depression but he can explain the supposed neurochemical mechanism that causes depression. Patients routinely report the results of lab tests, their diagnoses, and the dosages of drugs they take, but they struggle to describe their actual symptoms.

We have become so wrapped up in theory and explanation that we have lost the ability to simply acknowledge *what is*. We have lost touch with direct experience. This is what I refer to as *the death of experience*. It is the hallmark of our time. As a culture, we have become adept at overriding experiential reality in favor of the latest theories proposed by the sciences.

The death of experience inevitably leads to devaluation of personal knowledge, which in turn leads to both loss of personal autonomy and greater reliance upon external sources of authority. A parent learns, therefore, to ignore intuition and accepts the doctor's reassurances, allowing her daughter to be vaccinated for the umpteenth time, in disregard of the fact that she ran a high fever and became very ill after the last vaccination.

Medicine is not the only factor responsible for the death of experience. We can spend time alone in our living spaces, sometimes for days, without once stepping foot outside. We have television and computers to occupy and pacify our minds. We don't need to know the position of the sun in the sky because we have clocks to tell us the time of day. We travel in encapsulated vehicles, protected from the elements. We communicate via technology, sometimes never seeing friends or family for years on end. Modern civilization is decidedly insulated from nature. And the further we are from nature, the further we get from ourselves.

We drink coffee to wake up, alcohol to relax at the end of the day, and take pills to fall asleep. It is fair to say that society has adopted an anesthetic approach to life. We have a smorgasbord of pills to blot out anxiety, anger, sadness, and all forms of physical discomfort. Modern medicine is but a reflection of modern culture, which encourages us to live in a chronic state of avoidance, isolated from humanity, insulated from nature, in a diminished state of awareness, anesthetized from suffering, and in a pervasive state of denial regarding many aspects of our lives. Both medicine and culture share the same basic coping strategy—and that strategy is suppression.

As we slowly sink into an anesthetic haze, we increasingly turn responsibility for our lives over to persons and entities other than ourselves. In essence, we exchange ownership of personal experience for the false promise of comfort and security. Once the transfer has been made, and the "experts" are in control, not only do those promises ring hollow, but it also becomes increasingly difficult to take control of our lives once again.

The outcome of so much dissociation and denial must inevitably be compromised health. Not only do we not know how we feel or what it is that is wrong with us, but we have also ceded control of potential solutions to outside forces whose objectives do not necessarily coincide with our best interests.

Which brings us back to homeopathy. After all, it is not necessary to surrender to the depersonalizing nature of Western medicine. There are viable alternatives and, in my opinion, homeopathy is the most complete and effective alternative. Homeopathy is radical precisely because it is an experience-based system of healing that ultimately leads back to self-knowledge and self-empowerment. One cannot undertake homeopathic treatment without becoming more aware of mind and body. In the homeopathic world, experience is primary, and personal experience points the way toward healing.

A homeopathic practitioner is not interested in a patient's experience of illness just because he or she is trying to project an image of caring. Patient's descriptions and interpretations of their illnesses are required information without which the prospect of healing is unlikely. Patient and healer together must dig deep in order to read between the lines, in the hope of discovering a real solution, not just another pill to temporarily numb the pain.

Homeopathy is a powerful antidote to the anesthetic life. Homeopathy is a threat to any medical system that requires submission to a materialist agenda. While suppression ensures that patients remain dulled and dissociated, homeopathic healing promotes greater awareness and autonomy. With awareness comes greater personal responsibility. It also offers the potential for greater fulfillment and the freedom to experience life again to the fullest extent possible. Homeopathy is revolutionary because it offers a radical alternative to modern medicine and our anesthetized way of life.

Everything that we need to heal the planet is already at our disposal

Literally any substance is a potential healing agent. Think about that for a moment. Once transformed into their homeopathic essences, all substances of plant, mineral, and animal origin have the capacity to heal. It doesn't matter whether those substances are toxic or benign; they can be safely used as medicines once their energetic properties have been harnessed and studied. The few thousand medicines in the current homeopathic pharmacy are just drops in the bucket compared to the multitude of healing agents that nature can potentially provide.

Although some homeopathic medicines are made from highly toxic substances (arsenic, mercury, snake venom, spider venom, etc.), their extremely low dosages render them completely safe. It is literally impossible to be poisoned by a properly prepared homeopathic remedy.

Homeopathic medicines are also remarkably inexpensive. Since the substances found in nature used to make homeopathic medicines cannot be patented unless they are somehow chemically or structurally altered, PhRMA has no interest in exploiting them for profit. This among other reasons allows homeopathic pharmacies to keep the costs of production consistently low.

Furthermore, no matter how rare a homeopathic raw material is, there will always be an abundance of it available in homeopathic form. This is made possible by the homeopathic manufacturing process, which requires only a tiny amount of an original substance in order to convert it into millions of doses of potentized medicine. This should be of particular comfort to all who are concerned about animal welfare and environmental health. It sounds incredible but it requires only one honeybee to sacrifice its life in order to make enough *Apis mellifica* to meet the needs of the entire human population for decades to come. Given its breadth of application to human illness and its power to heal, homeopathy is about as ecofriendly as a system of healing can be. There is no animal testing or need for synthetic chemicals in any phase of production of homeopathic medicines.

It should be noted that although this book concerns itself with the treatment of human illness, veterinarians have used homeopathy for many decades to successfully treat the entire spectrum of animal illnesses. Small animal or large, it makes no difference. The very same principles used to treat human illness are equally effective when applied to animals.

Amazingly, homeopathy is also used with great success in agriculture. Agrohomeopathy is a specialized field that concerns itself with the health of plants and soils. It has practical applications that are invaluable in farming, horticulture, arboriculture, floriculture, and even soil science. This basic truth regarding the broad applicability of homeopathy should be enough to pique the interest of any truly inquisitive person—and even a few skeptics.

And if the fact that homeopathy is safe, effective, inexpensive, and broadly applicable to all life on the planet were not enough, there is one more very important point worth noting. Dr. Kent alludes to that point in the quote at the start of this chapter. Everything that we need to heal the planet is already at our disposal. Nature contains within it all that is needed to heal all life forms. Homeopathy is simply a tool that allows us to tap into a healing power that already exists in nature.

Homeopathy is in its relative infancy. Given time, adequate resources, and the human will to accomplish the task, many thousands more medicines could be made and properly studied; medicines that could heal virtually all forms of illness on the planet. Given the immense resistance from orthodox medicine that it has faced throughout its short 200-year life span, homeopathy has just scratched the surface of its enormous potential. Homeopathy has spread across the globe against all odds. Imagine what could be accomplished with a little support and cooperation.

Now, there is one important caveat to this admittedly idealistic vision of healing. Nature is no longer what she once was. For many decades nature has been systematically exploited and polluted by modern man, in particular by science and industry. Nature has become a vast dumping ground for untold numbers of synthetic substances. I'll never forget an ecology class that I took back in college. The professor told us about a study that examined the chemical composition of oysters dredged up from the bottom of the Chesapeake Bay. Spectrographic analysis identified literally hundreds of man-made chemical compounds in those oysters, some of which were identifiable and others that were not. And it's scary to think that that study was conducted back in the early 1970s.

Given the extent to which nature has been tainted, the toxicity and carcinogenicity of many synthetic substances, and the unknown effects of many others, it is not hard to see how profoundly this would impact not only human health but the health of the entire ecosystem and all the life forms that depend upon it. Add to this chemical soup a new generation of GMOs and nanotech substances courtesy of the biotech industry, and it is not surprising that new, previously unknown manmade diseases would spring up from this ungodly swamp created by scientific progress.

In principle, homeopathy renders most synthetic drugs obsolete. However, with the introduction of synthetic chemicals, new forms of unnatural illness can occasionally require unnatural treatment. A homeopathic preparation of a synthetic drug may help heal a person who suffers from the effects of having taken that drug in its pharmaceutical form. For example, it would be reasonable to treat a person who had psychological problems after a bad LSD trip by administering homeopathic doses of LSD. At the very least, the chemical and pharmaceutical industries have made the successful treatment of human illness a good bit more complicated.

Given that caveat, *almost* everything we need for healing is within reach. It makes perfect sense that nature would contain within it all that is needed to heal human illness. Why would it be any other way? It violates basic common sense to think that humankind would be placed on this planet having to synthesize an endless string of highly toxic substances in order to heal its wounds. On the other hand, it makes perfect sense that a civilization cut off from nature would seek unnatural, artificial solutions to its health problems.

Although humanity is but a reflection of nature, modern man seems to think he is exempt from this basic reality. Western civilization has isolated itself from nature to such an extent that one can easily be deluded into thinking that it is possible to exist independently from nature. Nothing could be further from the truth. This belief cuts to the very heart of the spiritual sickness of modern man. He mistakenly and arrogantly sees himself as manipulator of nature and controller of his own destiny.

Radical healing

By now it should be clear that homeopathy is both revolutionary and subversive. Those who experience successful homeopathic treatment are often changed in ways that they could not have anticipated. When we begin to question how it is possible that homeopathy can work at all, it profoundly alters our perception of the world around us. Once the implications of homeopathic treatment sink in, one cannot help but see things from a completely different perspective, from a radically different paradigm than that of mainstream science and medicine.

Homeopathy is controversial because it challenges some of our most cherished beliefs and values. It changes our understanding of mind and body. It flies in the face of body-centered materialistic medicine. Homeopathy does not simply acknowledge the reality of mind. It confirms over and over that mind and body are one. Even the term *mindbody* is misleading. It does not mean that mind and body are two separate but interconnected things. Mind and body are one and the same.

Just to be clear, it's not that all is mind, or that all is in the mind. All is mindbody, with health disturbances manifesting to varying degrees as physical, mental, emotional, or spiritual symptomatology. Perhaps it is more complete to say that all is *bodyheartmindsoul*.

Mindbody is just a convenient but artificial term used to refer to an idea that is foreign to those who interpret life and illness from the concrete three-dimensional paradigm of mainstream medicine. It is hard enough for scientists to believe that there is such a thing as mind, let alone the idea that mind and body are the same.

The consensus view of modern science is that mind is an "epiphenomenon," a mere byproduct of brain neurochemistry. Science's materialist bias prevents it from considering the possibility that the brain, like a radio that channels radio waves, could be a receiver and transmitter of consciousness. Three-dimensional medicine is not ready to admit the existence of a fourth dimension. But without the fourth dimension of consciousness, without a life force to organize and maintain homeostasis, the human body would be nothing more than an amorphous soup.

Homeopathy demonstrates in practical terms the energetic nature of all things. All is one and all is energy. That which we call matter is just a more dense and compact manifestation of energy. Einstein's theory of special relativity demonstrates the idea of mass-energy equivalence, which is to say that mass is nothing more than concentrated energy. That is why it is possible to say that body and mind are the same. All phenomena, material and immaterial, are manifestations of energy along a continuum. Mainstream science conceptualizes energy from the lowest frequency radio waves to the highest frequency gamma rays. But it fails to incorporate matter on the low end of the spectrum and mind at the higher end.

Call it mind, call it consciousness, or energy, or chi, or spirit, or the life force; it doesn't really matter. All are legitimate terms that refer to a mysterious fourth dimension, a dimension that science and medicine mistakenly dismiss as irrelevant to health and healing. We live in a unified universe where all things vibrate at their own unique frequencies.

We can acknowledge this reality, take the time to study its properties and principles, and make use of this valuable knowledge for the betterment of humankind, or we can go on as we have, digging ourselves deeper into the materialistic muck with the help of mainstream medicine. We can work with the life force or we can work against it. The choice is ours.

The vibratory frequency of the life force changes when it experiences distress, resulting in a distinct pattern of symptoms. Each homeopathic remedy has a unique energy frequency, which can be identified by the symptom pattern that it can cause. When matching energy signatures of remedy and sick individual are brought together, which is to say, when the two frequencies resonate, it creates a type of constructive interference that resolves the dysfunction of the vital force thus returning it to energetic balance, to its previously healthy baseline state.

Homeopathy is revolutionary because it changes the very nature and purpose of medicine itself. The goal is not just to relieve pain or discomfort; it is to restore health and balance. The goal is not just to suppress symptoms; it is to peel back the layers, to unravel the cumulative dysfunction of the life force. The goal is not just physical health; homeopathy's aim is the health of body, heart, mind, and soul. Although such expectations are far higher than orthodox medicine could ever dream of, they are not unrealistic. Our expectations regarding allopathic medicine are remarkably low. We tend to accept increasingly greater risks for only modest benefits. Homeopathic treatment may not always achieve its lofty agenda but, when it does, it is a truly remarkable thing to behold.

Homeopathy accomplishes all this without generating nasty side effects, without the need for synthetic substances, without poisoning the environment with those substances, and without doing harm to animals. And to top it all off, homeopathy reduces the likelihood of price gouging and corporate exploitation.

As if that were not enough, homeopathy also serves as a tool for conscious evolution. In other words, it is a healing modality that, when practiced with skill, tends to promote growth of consciousness. I don't mean the slow, cruel, random kind of survival-of-the-fittest Darwinian evolution that we have all been taught courtesy of materialist science. Homeopathy facilitates a more immediate type of psycho-spiritual evolution that manifests itself as greater awareness, emotional balance and maturity, and spiritual receptivity.

To me, illness is blocked energy, the consequence of which is arrested development. Chronic illness that refuses to yield is indicative of obstructed consciousness. This is the reason why so many people learn valuable life lessons through the suffering that accompanies illness. The obstruction is only meant to be temporary, just long enough to absorb the message hiding within it. Note that this is not the same as saying that people cause their own illnesses or have the voluntary power to think their way out of their illnesses. Illness is very complex and often beyond our control. That's why chronic illness is chronic. It defies our ability to solve it on our own. Sometimes the lesson is as simple as learning how to ask for help.

Homeopathy can radically alter the course of people's lives by releasing them from the energetic grip of their illnesses. When the vital force is no longer preoccupied with illness it can be redirected toward higher purposes of personal growth and service to humanity. Consciousness and illness are just positive and negative sides of the same coin. Illness is the spur that holds the key to healing and its consequent increase of awareness. I've seen cosmic doors open more than a few times after my patients have received the correct remedy. It's as if the universe recognizes that the situation has changed for the better, thus allowing opportunities for growth and advancement to materialize in unexpected ways—opportunities that the person would have been unable to take advantage of in his or her prior state of ill health. I am often left to wonder what a particular patient's life would have been like had he or she not received that much-needed remedy.

The uniquely empowering benefits of homeopathy are especially apparent in children whose lives can turn on a dime after receiving a well-chosen remedy. By altering a child's negative health trajectory early on, a great deal of unnecessary suffering can be avoided. Western medicine has led many to conclude that there is nothing that can be done about what are perceived to be the inalterable "personality traits" of some children who exhibit difficult or problematic behaviors. One parent is inclined to throw up his hands in resignation when his son throws yet another temper tantrum after losing the ball game, writing it off to his "competitive nature." Another parent learns to accept that the inhibited behavior of her son is a function of his "sensitive nature."

But homeopaths know that these so-called personality traits are really not traits as much as they are symptomatic exaggerations, deviations from the norm that can be moderated by good homeopathic care. Even when told of homeopathy's potential to help such problems, most don't believe it. It sounds too good to be true. Nevertheless, I remain hopeful that homeopathy will someday be recognized for the role that it can play as a powerful form of developmental medicine.

Some can get a little freaked out when they hear homeopaths talk like this. They worry that homeopathy is some strange form of mind control or social engineering. They may compare it to psychiatric drugs, which, after all, do constitute a type of chemical control over behavior. Of course, nothing could be further from the truth. Either a homeopathic remedy fits or it doesn't. If it doesn't fit, it won't work. And when it works, it only works in the sense that it restores the life force to balance. Unless it is abused and taken on a prolonged basis, no homeopathic remedy can impose an unwanted state upon a person.

Homeopathy is less of an analytic approach than it is a phenomenological approach. It concerns itself with *what is* rather than *why it is*. Homeopathy is more descriptive than explanatory. Hahnemann rightly warned against speculative explanations regarding disease causation. He understood that such explanations were fraught with bias and error. He also understood that the lack of effective therapeutic options available to orthodox physicians left them with nothing to do but speculate endlessly over the causes of disease.

Descriptions of states of illness, on the other hand, are what they are. They are not subject to debate. Homeopathy takes a patient's description of his or her symptoms at face value and seeks a homeopathic medicine to match those symptoms. This approach to healing challenges our very concept of what it is that makes medicine scientific. While medicine busies itself with trying to determine the name and cause of an illness, homeopathy can effectively bypass those steps while proceeding directly to treatment. This doesn't preclude the fact that a good homeopath turns to diagnostics when necessary and also knows how to read between the lines in order to discern unspoken issues that may be contributing to an illness.

Cultural programming can be hard to overcome. Most people want explanations for their illnesses. Of course, explanations wouldn't really matter that much if medicine could provide real relief from chronic illness. Patients are conditioned, instead, to accept scholarly sounding discourses couched in scientific lingo in lieu of successful treatment. We are dazzled by medical jargon, which serves to temporarily distract us from the reality that there are no satisfactory solutions for most chronic diseases. Here, again, we see why modern medicine is best characterized as *rational*, while homeopathy is best described as *empirical*. In the best of all worlds, the two approaches together would make a formidable system of medical healing.

Homeopathy is revolutionary because it subverts the homogenized nature of medical culture. It defies one-size-fits-all diagnosis and treatment by demanding that attention be given to the uniqueness of each suffering individual and his or her illness. In doing so, it reasserts the primacy of patient experience. All the stats and research studies don't amount to much if they fail to provide individualized solutions for each and every suffering person. Homeopathy does not pigeonhole patients and their illnesses. There are no shortcuts that allow a homeopathic practitioner to dispense with the hard work of taking a patient's case and searching for the *simillimum*.

Homeopathy replaces the fragmented worldview of mainstream medicine with a truly holistic vision of interconnectedness. A symptom is neither random nor meaningless, and is always connected, whether by space, time, or significance, in some way to all other symptoms and problems. One cannot treat a part without impacting the whole, even if that impact is not always discernable. While specialized medicine may be technically proficient, it is also several steps removed from holistic reality and can, as a result, produce unintended consequences somewhere along the mindbody continuum. Homeopathy, by contrast, is always cognizant of the overall direction of healing. It cannot be considered healing when one part improves while another, more vital part, worsens. True holism accounts for all aspects of the sick person.

Homeopathy does not resort to facile gimmicks as a substitute for healing. It is not acceptable to attribute the ubiquitous but nebulous phenomenon of *stress* for all the problems that medicine cannot solve. We can do better that that; homeopathy does do better than that. Stress has become a scapegoat for all that orthodox medicine cannot explain. It is incapable of understanding the true nature of stress, thanks to its failure to acknowledge the mind-body connection and the role of consciousness in illness. After all, what is stress other than the effects of mind upon body?

Homeopathy has no such problem understanding mind-body interactions. It excels at treating stress-related problems, which I dare say constitute the majority of human illnesses. It never occurs to orthodox medical thinkers that stress is not just a cause of illness; it is also a result. This explains why persons of good health can withstand similar stressors far better than those in poor health. I often find myself having to reassure patients that homeopathy should be able to restore their health in spite of the perceived stressors.

Unlike mainstream medicine, homeopathy is both unchanging and enduring. Its foundational principle remains the same. The symptoms that any given substance can cause remain the same. The symptom patterns of human illness are also the same as they were a hundred years ago. The only thing that changes is the homeopathic armamentarium. The number of remedies available for homeopathic use grows with each passing decade.

By contrast, allopathy is inherently unstable. It's theories, medicines, and protocols change on a regular basis. The true reason for this is its flawed and incomplete understanding of health and illness. Its materialist perspective and reductionist approach will always fall short of holistic reality. Since its foundational beliefs are incorrect, its strategies for treating illness must, of necessity, be ever changing.

While mainstream medicine has a distinctly paternalistic streak, homeopathy is remarkably egalitarian. A good homeopath can't afford to tell the patient what to do and what to think. He or she must listen very carefully to everything the patient has to say, knowing that some clue that leads to therapeutic success may be revealed at any moment. It is a collaborative process by which patient and practitioner are constantly learning from their experiences and interactions. Doctor teaches patient and patient teaches doctor.

By taking patients and their concerns seriously, homeopathy also has the net overall effect of diminishing the stigma attached to their conditions. Whether the problem is hypochondria, hysteria, herpes, a sexually transmitted infection, or just plain old lack of self-confidence, homeopathy does not make value judgments regarding such problems. It seeks to understand them in order to heal them.

Homeopathy is based on a principle, not a philosophy. The principle of similars has been observed over and over both in nature and in the clinic. Whether we consider it a law of nature is a question for debate. Hahnemann used the principle of similars to fashion a system of healing, out of which emerged a philosophical perspective regarding the nature of health, illness, and healing. That philosophy is kept honest by consistently checking its assertions against actual clinical outcomes.

When we witness or experience the amazing results of homeopathic treatment, it cannot but alter our understanding of the nature of life itself. That understanding is radically different from the worldview engendered by the allopathic medical perspective. I am well acquainted with the sense of awe provided by the revelations that come with the experience of homeopathic transformation. The lessons taught by homeopathy are both humbling and inspiring. It is a sentiment that is far from new, as is made clear when one reads the words of one of our great homeopathic forebears, Charles J. Hempel, MD—words that were written over a century and a half ago. I can assure you that the feeling is mutual:

> *If I have succeeded in showing that the science of homœopathy is as liberal and progressive as Nature; that it is a truth not belonging to any one man, or set of men, but that it is heaven-born, resting upon eternal foundations, shedding its vitalizing rays over all minds and enlightening each according to the measure of his capacity: I shall believe that I have done our cause some service.*[78]

A word about homeopathic politics

Even though homeopathy has been around for two hundred years, it is still only in its infancy. During that time it has met with a great deal of resistance from the dominant school of medicine. Homeopathy rose up, reached its peak in the late 1800s, subsequently declined, and has been on the rise again over the last fifty years. Its survival in the face of so much adversity is a testament to its power to heal.

One can only imagine what homeopathy might have achieved if it did not have to contend with constant threats to its survival. Where would it be if it had actual support from government, the medical mainstream, and other public institutions? No doubt, the status of homeopathy would be significantly different than it is today.

Nevertheless it has flourished, albeit with scant resources. Homeopathy has prospered thanks to the dedication of many courageous individuals. Believe me, advocating for homeopathy is not for the weak-kneed. It takes a special kind of fortitude, an ability to withstand cultural criticism and social disapproval. It oftentimes means that one must live an isolated professional life without the local support of like-minded colleagues.

For this reason, homeopathy tends to attract strong-minded individuals who are willing to stand up for what is right, even in the face of opposition. One can imagine what it must be like when groups of such individuals get together to form societies dedicated to homeopathy. One might think that it is not much different from mainstream medical culture, which is similarly populated by ambitious and driven individuals. Well yes, and no. Conventional physicians are content with the way things are. They do not look to challenge the status quo. Homeopaths, on the other hand, can be a contentious lot because they tend to be mavericks. Even if they are in agreement regarding homeopathy, they can still disagree about almost everything else.

Now add to this the fact that homeopathy is so remarkably effective. Its ability to heal is unparalleled, so much so that it is a quantum leap or two beyond all other healing modalities. Of course, no one other than homeopaths and their patients know this. Everyone else thinks it's just another holistic therapy. Most people don't even know what homeopathy is; they mistakenly think it's herbal or nutritional medicine.

When the average person experiences the healing power of homeopathy firsthand, it can be a transformative moment. It is only natural that newcomers would be inspired to tell family and friends about this new discovery. To their surprise, however, new converts are often dismayed at the skepticism they encounter when sharing the good news. It's enough to cause some to censor themselves, to keep their healing secret quiet.

On the other hand, strong-minded mavericks who encounter the healing power of homeopathy are not likely to be deterred by resistance. In fact, they may go a little overboard, tending to overstate the case. Let's face it; the effectiveness of homeopathy can be intoxicating and inspiring. Given the fact that all else pales in comparison, true believers can be a little zealous in their estimation of homeopathy's benefits. I am not criticizing the enthusiasm of newcomers; it is only natural. But it can occasionally lead to problems.

Homeopathic success can be seductive and may lead to high expectations. Once you've seen it work, it is easy to think that it can cure anything. Those new to homeopathy can be very idealistic. It engenders high standards and may cause one to become critical of conventional medicine, which, after all, by contrast is like using an old fashioned typewriter to write a book. Practitioners new to homeopathy can sometimes make outlandish claims. Even some well-established homeopaths have been known to state that they can cure complex illnesses like autism, cancer, or schizophrenia. While such claims may occasionally be true, oftentimes they are not. It is best to be wary of the practitioner who makes such unqualified claims.

While the potential is there for homeopathy to be able to heal just about everything under the sun, the day-to-day reality of dealing with sick patients can bring the idealist back down to earth. It is easy for the practitioner to assume that the right remedy can solve any problem. However, it requires a great deal of knowledge and experience to be able to choose a correct remedy. And in spite of all the knowledge in the world, the needed remedy may have yet to be proven and may not be found in the *materia medica*.

It should come as no surprise, then, when newcomers discover that there are so many factions and disputes within homeopathy's ranks. I like to think of homeopathy as the holistic Wild West of medicine, that forbidden frontier where few dare to tread. The courageous few are out there blazing trails and panning for gold but sometimes those trails lead to dead ends, and some prospectors may find only fool's gold.

But that is to be expected. All lines of inquiry do not necessarily lead to success. We can only admire those healing pioneers for trying.

While most homeopaths are in agreement with Hahnemann's principle of similars, differences can arise over a variety of ancillary issues. One broad category of disagreement has to do with the best way to administer remedies. Homeopaths often disagree over remedy potency and frequency of dosing. Classical homeopaths insist that only one remedy at a time should be given. Others practice polypharmacy, which involves the prescribing of multiple remedies concurrently. This practice deviates from Hahnemann's original ideal and is largely influenced by the reductionist thinking typical of orthodox medicine. It is, in essence, a misguided form of allopathic homeopathy.

Although I have always disliked labels, I subscribe mostly to the classical school of homeopathy. I prescribe single remedies at long intervals, except in the event of unusual circumstances. I use a wide range of potencies and tend to believe that disputes over potency are a waste of time. Remedy potency is not nearly as important as choosing the correct remedy. The correct remedy will often work well regardless of the potency used. For this reason, I suspect that potency disputes are a distraction from the fact that the correct remedy can be difficult to determine. It's easier to blame the wrong potency for one's lack of success than to admit that choosing the homeopathic *simillimum* is challenging work.

Historically, there was an unfortunate dispute between high and low-dose schools of prescribing. Because of their high degree of dilution, some of the more conventionally minded homeopaths didn't believe that high potency remedies could possibly work. High potency prescribers eventually came to be thought of as quacks by low potency prescribers who considered themselves more scientific. Most modern homeopaths do not doubt the power of high potency prescribing. The high-low schism was one factor that kept homeopaths from unifying effectively in the face of allopathic opposition.

Another broad category of disagreement has to do with case analysis. Few homeopaths dispute the principle of similars, and all agree that patient's symptoms must be the primary guide to the choice of remedy. However, it turns out that there are many ways to analyze symptoms. Different methods of analysis will naturally tend to yield different remedy choices. Herein lies the cutting edge of contemporary homeopathy.

Such differences are both legitimate and desirable. They constitute different approaches in the quest for the correct remedy. There is a great deal of creative ferment and innovative thinking when it comes to case analysis. It's a good thing for homeopaths to experiment with new methods. It's reasonable to assume that the more successful methods will endure while less productive strategies will fall to the wayside.

Certain critics like to point to the chaotic profusion of homeopathic ideas as evidence of its unscientific nature. I actually believe that the reverse it true. It suggests that homeopathy is a field of great scientific ferment. Homeopathy is a dynamic method of healing with an evolving body of knowledge, the full potential of which has barely been tapped. The future of homeopathy is very bright indeed. Contrast this with the deep sense of settled certainty of allopathic medicine, which is more an indication of closed-mindedness than conviction.

Now there is one particular aspect of homeopathic politics that does concern me. I alluded to this point earlier. The intoxicating effect of homeopathic success can combine with the ambitious nature of some individuals to make for a toxic mix. While that mix may fuel innovation, it also creates a homeopathic frontier where some ego-driven individuals can be motivated by the quest for personal aggrandizement. A few are inclined to insist that their way is the best way. They like to attach their names to their "discoveries" as if it is acceptable for such knowledge to be owned exclusively. They fancy themselves as the latest gurus on the homeopathic scene.

Such misleading and unscrupulous claims would be easy to overlook if it weren't for unsuspecting newcomers who are inclined to fall for the hype. The world is full of people who are far too willing to follow leaders. There is no shortage of individuals who believe that their guru's way is the only way. For this reason, I reject the commonly used designation, "master homeopath." It runs counter to the egalitarian spirit of true homeopathic collaboration. I accept the term when used as an honorary title to refer to Dr. Hahnemann himself. When used otherwise, it undermines homeopathic collegiality and the sharing of ideas, and gives some the impression that select individuals possess secrets that others do not.

For similar reasons, I dislike the use of the word "cure" in homeopathic discourse. It carries with it an unrealistic connotation of finality. I much prefer to speak of the "direction of healing." It is provisional and less certain, less sure of itself. It acknowledges the fact that healing is an ongoing process that is never fully completed. Although homeopathy is certainly curative in comparison to allopathy in general, as far as I am concerned, it still sends the wrong message.

Personally, I am a purist. I believe that the collective work of the homeopathic community must be kept in the public domain. In modern terminology, it should always remain open source. The great magnum opus of homeopathic healing is far too important to be owned, even in part, by any one person. The fact that homeopathic medicines cannot be patented is a built-in advantage that serves homeopathy well. The day homeopathy becomes a commodity is the day that it becomes true snake oil, no better than the latest pharmaceutical "miracle" drug. Homeopathy is God's great healing gift to humanity. It must not be allowed to be defiled by the petty desires of the human ego.

Back to the future

There is no telling how much suffering homeopathy could relieve if it were given the resources and support that it deserves. Only time will tell. As the popularity of homeopathy continues to grow there is one particular issue that will be critical to its long-term survival. It must be able to maintain its methodological integrity in the face of pressure to become more modern and "scientific."

Western medicine has a way of undermining alternative healing methods that do not conform to its way of seeing things. When something like yoga, for example, manages to maintain its popularity in spite of attempts to discredit it, medicine changes tactics, trying instead to make it its own. All sorts of relaxation methods suddenly crop up in medical settings, giving the impression that medicine has somehow "discovered" a new stress relieving technique that it now markets as a holistic gimmick to its patients.

This wouldn't be so bad if it didn't have the effect of diluting true yoga down to a mere caricature. Patients who think they are being taught yoga wind up learning a few postures and stretching exercises, which together constitute a shadow of the full healing potential that a serious commitment to yoga could provide. Medicine assimilates what it wants for its own purposes, the rest is rejected, and patients are none the wiser.

Homeopathy has already been through that ringer before. Low potency prescribing was taken somewhat seriously for a brief period in history (primarily by allopathically minded physicians), the rest was dismissed, and the integrity of homeopathy suffered, thus leading to its near extinction. If homeopathy is to rise to prominence once again, it is imperative that it not allow itself to be destroyed by allopathic propaganda campaigns that paint it as unscientific. While homeopathy may not be scientific in a way that satisfies conventional medicine's litmus test, it is highly scientific in its own right and in its own unique way. It is scientific in ways that make orthodox medicine look comparatively archaic.

It is incumbent upon the homeopathic community to be vigilant so that history does not repeat itself. When it approaches critical mass, homeopathy will begin to achieve popular acclaim. Having failed to sabotage homeopathy, mainstream medicine will then attempt to co-opt it as if it were its own. When it goes mainstream homeopathy will be pressured to conform to allopathic expectation and, if it does, it will be mangled beyond recognition. If orthodoxy succeeds in assimilating homeopathy, it will surely be reduced to an impotent shadow of its former self, thus assuring that it is relegated to historical oblivion once again.

Whenever conventional medicine tries to superimpose its conceptual framework on homeopathy the outcome is always disappointing. This is why conventional research trials fail to do justice to the true power of homeopathy. In their current configuration, such trials are fundamentally incompatible with homeopathic methodology and do not yield information that leads to any greater understanding. While medicine presumptuously demands proof of the efficacy of homeopathy in abstract statistical terms, it conveniently ignores the countless thousands of positive clinical outcomes documented by physicians over the past two hundred years. Medicine pigheadedly refuses to accept personal experience as a valid form of evidence.

Likewise, when orthodox medicine assumes it can apply a this-for-that mentality to homeopathic prescribing, it completely misses the mark. Homeopathy is the very antithesis of cookie-cutter medicine. Homeopathy cannot be assimilated into an allopathic milieu without losing its integrity as a holistic discipline. It must be accepted on its own terms and allowed to stand side by side with conventional medicine. Only then will its true potential be realized.

I happen to believe that neither biology, nor chemistry, nor physics will ever be able to explain homeopathy. All are reductionist sciences and no reductionist science can ever give a full accounting of any holistic phenomenon. While homeopathy does work its magic with the help of biology, chemistry, and physics, it also operates at a more profound level. Call it energy, spirit, consciousness, or the life force; the materialist metaphysics of conventional science will never be able to grasp its true significance. Homeopathy can only be understood through the lens of a more comprehensive and enlightened paradigm.

If there is hope for the salvation of humankind it is to be found in the dynamic healing power of homeopathy. Homeopathy doesn't always work but, boy, when it does it is truly amazing. What else could possibly repair the deepest wounds of the human psyche, wounds that often lie at the roots of our physical ailments? What else can neutralize the deleterious impact of generations of inherited dysfunction? What else can simultaneously heal the planet without poisoning the planet?

What else costs pennies to produce and can be distributed across the globe at minimal expense? Nothing, of course. Only homeopathy can do those things. And if you don't believe me, you should try it for yourself!

Appendix of Practical Homeopathic Tips

Choosing a homeopathic practitioner

In order to ensure a positive healing experience, it is important that one carefully choose a homeopathic practitioner. Given the nature of the homeopathic Wild West, it is important to understand that some who claim to practice homeopathy are, in actuality, not really homeopaths. Some are dabblers who know little about homeopathy. Some purchase an array of combination remedies and prescribe by number, according to the indications on the labels. Others use homeopathy as an afterthought, just another option in their wide array of holistic offerings.

Classical homeopathy is the style of homeopathy that remains most faithful to Hahnemann's original method. I believe it is best suited to achieving the most successful outcomes. A good classical homeopath must spend an adequate amount of time—anywhere from ninety minutes to two or more hours on the first visit—in order to gather the information needed to provide quality care. With rare exceptions, a classical homeopath prescribes only one homeopathic medicine at a time. A good homeopath also knows that it is important to give adequate time in between remedy prescriptions. Given circumstances, this can mean waiting up to three or four weeks and sometimes months before another dose of remedy is recommended.

Any practitioner that fails to spend the time needed to get to know his or her patients, or prescribes multiple remedies in quick succession, is not observing the fundamental principles of classical homeopathic care. It is easy to determine the nature of a homeopath's practice by asking questions about whether he or she adheres to these classical principles.

There are two broad categories of homeopathic practitioners: those who have formal conventional medical training and those who do not. In addition to their homeopathic education, medically trained homeopaths have some type of conventional medical training. These medically trained homeopaths include medical doctors, osteopathic doctors, naturopathic doctors, veterinarians, dentists, physician assistants, nurse practitioners, registered nurses, acupuncturists, and chiropractors. Non-medical homeopaths who do not have medically related degrees, but who do have formal homeopathic training are also known as *professional homeopaths*.

Whether a practitioner is medically or non-medically trained is not necessarily an indication of homeopathic competence. It can be an important issue for some patients who would prefer a homeopath with a medical background. For others, it is the quality of homeopathic training that matters most. The quality of homeopathic training has nothing to do with whether one is medically trained or not. The bottom line is that there are good medical homeopaths and there are good professional homeopaths.

A good homeopath is not opposed to all things having to do with conventional medicine. A good homeopath knows when to refer his or her patients to a primary care physician or a specialist. Perhaps one of the main advantages of medically trained homeopaths is they can serve as mediators between their patients and the medical system. It is not uncommon for me to recommend that patients consult their allopathic doctors. Information provided by allopathic consultations can contribute to greater understanding of patients' health concerns and can help me make proper decisions regarding their homeopathic and allopathic care. A good homeopath is a good holistic health advocate.

A good practitioner respects patients' wishes and choices, even when he or she is not in agreement with those choices. It is best to avoid paternalistic practitioners who presume to know what is best for their patients and whose behavior can make patients feel bad or guilty about the decisions that they make. As mentioned earlier, the power of homeopathy can be intoxicating and may lead some to think that no health problem is insurmountable. It is natural for new practitioners to be enthusiastic about that potential. Their newfound passion may incline them to overstate the case, to criticize allopathic medicine, and to pressure patients to follow only their homeopathic advice. It is best to steer clear of practitioners who boast of their cured cases or offer guarantees of success.

I know; I was once that young, idealistic homeopathic doctor. I still have a passion for homeopathy, but I also know that people must be allowed to choose homeopathy of their own accord. No one should be coaxed or coerced into doing something that they have reservations about or feel reluctant to do. Patients have every right to disagree with my advice. I know that what I believe to be the right thing to do is not necessarily the right thing from the patient's perspective. The ideal relationship is one in which patient and practitioner work together with a mutual feeling of respect and trust.

Sometimes tension can arise when a patient's lack of ability or willingness to follow homeopathic protocol clashes with the prescriber's wishes to practice homeopathy according to the rulebook, so to speak. Different patients bring different degrees of understanding and commitment to the process. It is the practitioner's responsibility to educate patients about the homeopathic healing process. It is not reasonable for a practitioner to make unrealistic demands in the name of the purity of homeopathic principles. While there are rules that should be followed in order to maximize the probability of homeopathic success, those rules are really just guidelines. For example, while the goal should be less overall dependence on allopathic drugs, no practitioner has the right to demand that a patient discontinue taking all drugs at any point in the treatment process. A good homeopathic practitioner always remains flexible and is willing to adjust to the individual needs of his or her patients.

Basic guidelines to follow when under constitutional care

The first visit to a homeopathic practitioner will be an in-depth interview covering every aspect of the patient's health—physical, mental, and emotional. The patient should be prepared to give thoughtful answers no matter how seemingly tangential or unimportant a question may appear to be. However, spontaneity is also an important factor, so it is best not to prepare answers ahead of time.

Some people get excited after their first visit with a homeopath, run out and buy some remedies, and begin prescribing for themselves. This is not advisable. One should not treat oneself while under constitutional homeopathic care. Any remedy can potentially disrupt the effects of a previously taken remedy. It is best to inform the practitioner of any remedies taken other than the ones prescribed. If a problem arises that requires attention, it is preferable to contact one's caregiver rather than treat oneself. The treatment of chronic illness is especially complex. Best results are achieved when patient and practitioner are on the same page.

When first beginning homeopathic treatment, it can be difficult adjusting to a new way of dealing with illness. Old habits can be hard to break. Many are accustomed to taking over-the-counter (OTC) pills for runny noses, sneezing, headaches, and other minor symptoms. Moms may understandably feel that they don't want their children to suffer with such symptoms. It is up to the homeopathic doctor to explain why it is preferable to avoid most OTC drugs and how such a shortsighted symptomatic approach can lead to longer-term health problems.

Although most people are not accustomed to letting minor illnesses take their course, it is preferable to do so. It can instill a sense of confidence when one realizes that it is possible to recover from such problems on one's own without the help of drugs. A good practitioner knows that it is also not wise to give a homeopathic remedy for every little cough or cold. New symptoms can be a consequence of a previously taken remedy and may, therefore, be part of the natural healing process. On the other hand, when an illness is of concern, is too difficult to endure, or is not getting better on its own, it is best to contact your homeopathic caregiver.

The great antidoting debate

Those familiar with homeopathy are well acquainted with the concept of antidoting. *Antidotes* are certain factors that have the potential to prevent homeopathic remedies from doing their job. The most notorious antidoting factor is coffee. Many believe, as do I, that coffee can antidote the effects of remedies, even if a remedy was taken weeks or months earlier. I like to emphasize the point by telling my patients that coffee is "the kryptonite" of homeopathy. It is an apt metaphor because it paints a picture of one energy weakening the power of another energy. Not all homeopaths agree that coffee is an impediment to successful treatment. And as with kryptonite, not everyone is susceptible to coffee's antidoting effects.

Antidoting factors can cause varying degrees of disruption to the homeopathic healing process. An antidote can have a minor impact, causing a remedy to be less effective than it might otherwise have been. Sometimes an antidote can induce a complete relapse, erasing nearly all benefits of treatment up to that point.

The number of antidoting factors that homeopaths advise against has grown over the years. The list includes non-essential drugs, homeopathic remedies, all forms of coffee, including decaffeinated coffee and coffee flavored ice cream, and strong aromatic substances such and camphor, menthol, eucalyptus, and products that contain them. Medical procedures that involve anesthesia or sedation can also have an adverse impact on the action of homeopathic remedies. Dental work, drilling, and dental anesthesia can be antidoting factors. Likewise, x-rays, CT scans, and MRI scans are concentrated forms of energy that can disrupt the energetic effects of a remedy.

Since it is not always possible to avoid all antidoting factors, it is best to discuss the issue ahead of time with one's homeopathic practitioner. A reasonable homeopath will be willing to negotiate a sensible compromise. When I find out, for example, that my patient must have a cavity filled, I find ways to work around it. I may advise that the prescription be taken after the dental work is completed.

Giving up coffee can be a thorny issue for many java lovers. More than a few have forgone homeopathic care as a result. There is good reason why so many around the globe cannot do without their coffee. Coffee is a powerful and sometimes addictive substance. Some have the ability to discontinue drinking coffee without much trouble. However, when a person will not or cannot voluntarily stop drinking coffee, it may be a sign that there is an underlying problem. In many cases, coffee serves as a form of self-medication. Such individuals would do well to seek to homeopathic care.

To be clear, it is not the caffeine in coffee that poses the problem. Thankfully, caffeinated tea does not seem to have the same effect. Many patients are relieved to discover that although it would be to their advantage to avoid coffee, they can still drink tea if they wish.

Oftentimes, conventional drugs are unavoidable and, although they can make treatment more challenging, they do not necessarily preclude the possibility of successful homeopathic treatment. Each case is unique and should be discussed with the homeopathic doctor. Successful homeopathic treatment commonly enables patients to safely discontinue the use of many such drugs.

As with all things in the homeopathic community, not everyone is in agreement when it comes to the topic of antidoting factors. On one end of the spectrum, some even advise against mint toothpastes. On the other end, a few have no problem allowing their patients to drink coffee. As a physician, I feel ethically bound to advise my patients about potential antidotes. If a patient questions this or mentions some other homeopath who does not advise against coffee, for example, I explain that avoiding an antidote like coffee will increase the odds of successful treatment. It will ensure that his or her homeopathic experience was not a waste of time and money. For those who just can't give up coffee, I ask them to reduce their intake as much as possible in the hope that treatment will eventually enable them to kick the habit.

There is no doubt that the antidoting issue can be overplayed by some homeopaths. In such cases, I suspect that it is easier to blame patients and their antidoting indiscretions for poor outcomes rather than the practitioner's own inability to find the correct remedy for the person in question. Antidoting factors should not become an excuse for every time treatment fails to produce the desired results.

Homeopathic home-care for family and friends

Homeopathy spread across the early American frontier by virtue of the fact that mothers had access to remedy kits and first-aid literature. Homeopathy's reputation for success was slowly passed on by word of mouth from one family to another. And homeopathic self-care is still going strong today.

I must begin by making clear that no one should treat a condition at home that would normally compel one to seek professional help. Treatment of self-limiting conditions such as colds and minor injuries can be attempted at home. But treatment of serious acute illnesses and chronic conditions should always be left to a qualified practitioner. One should also not treat anyone who is already receiving professional homeopathic care. With that said, getting started is a simple matter of purchasing a few remedies and a few homeopathic first-aid books.

Countless homeopathy lovers became converts after witnessing the amazing healing power of *Arnica montana*. I recommend using *Arnica* for simple injuries as an entry point into first-aid homeopathy.[79] Start by purchasing a single bottle of *Arnica* 30c to use for minor injuries. *Arnica* is specifically indicated for soft tissue injuries that result in pain, soreness, bruising, swelling, and black and blue discoloration. Once convinced of the usefulness of *Arnica*, additional remedies can be purchased as situations arise.

There are a variety of homeopathic remedy kits on the market. It is best to start with a small kit of ten to thirty remedies for common conditions. The ideal potencies to use are 30x, 30D, 30c or 30CH. One can also use lower potencies. I do not recommend using higher potencies (200x, 200c, 1M, 10M, etc.) at home unless one has a lot of experience.

It is possible to purchase a larger kit at a later date after becoming more adept in the use of the remedies.

There are a good number of well-written first-aid books. Since different books provide slightly different perspectives about various health conditions and remedy possibilities, it is best to purchase several books to use as references. That way, for example, when a family member or friend sprains an ankle, one can read about sprains from several different sources before selecting a first-aid remedy.

One common problem is that enthusiastic newcomers without adequate knowledge or experience jump into homeopathy too quickly. It is preferable to start small and slowly work one's way up to more challenging first-aid situations. Another problem is that people naturally tend to view homeopathy from a conventional medical perspective. In other words, they tend to think they can use remedies like they use OTC drugs. There is a tendency to rely on them for every little sneeze or sniffle. There is great wisdom in allowing the body to work its problems out on its own. It is not always necessary to intervene with a drug or a remedy. Sometimes it is best to let nature take its course.

Another common mistake is to administer remedies repeatedly when it is not necessary. Again, remedies are not like drugs and, so, more is not necessarily better. Mild flu symptoms, for example, should respond quickly to a few doses of a remedy. If improvement is not apparent, it is not because more of the remedy is needed; it is because the wrong remedy has been chosen. It is preferable to go back to the reference books in search of another potential remedy choice.

Homeopathy is perfectly safe as long as one follows a few simple guidelines and puts the time and effort into learning about the remedies. By contrast, the use of conventional OTC drugs is far more hazardous. With a little time and effort it is possible to become a capable first-aid prescriber.

Using the medical system to your advantage

(Please note that most of what is discussed in this section applies to patients seeking care from homeopathic practitioners who also have conventional medical degrees.)

Successful homeopathic treatment often enables patients to discontinue taking their medications. Many seek homeopathic care specifically because they wish to avoid conventional drugs and their well-known side effects and dangers. But sometimes homeopathy works and sometimes it doesn't. In anticipation of therapeutic success, enthusiastic patients can sometimes discontinue taking their conventional drugs prematurely, even against the wishes of their homeopathic physicians. It is important to be realistic about the process.

Whether one should stop taking a drug or not, and how that can be done, are serious issues that should be discussed with one's homeopathic and conventional physicians. Some drugs are necessary and cannot be discontinued. Other drugs may be necessary in the short-run until patient's conditions improve enough to warrant discontinuation of their use. Every situation is unique and should be treated as such.

The medical system has its distinct advantages and weaknesses. Its therapeutic track record is particularly inadequate when it comes to the treatment of chronic disease. Homeopathy excels in the treatment of chronic disease. However, this does not mean that all pharmaceutical drugs are evil or to be avoided at all costs. Allopathic drugs can have their proper place in the scheme of things and should not be demonized.

Although diagnostic technology is conventional medicine's great strength, it too can be overused. As I have said before, medicine's obsession with diagnosis is a function of its therapeutic weakness. When patient's problems cannot be helped, it's easy to give the impression of doing something constructive by conducting additional tests or periodic tests to check on the status of those problems. Not infrequently, diagnostic testing has a tendency to confirm what was already known from the start. Sometimes it may be known ahead of time that the results of testing will not change the course of allopathic treatment. In some situations this kind of testing is warranted. Oftentimes it is not.

Although diagnostic technology has clear advantages, it also carries the potential for iatrogenic harm and can be overused when therapeutic options are limited. The challenge for patients is to determine when to consent to further testing and when to decline. Sometimes testing is well advised but sometimes it can expose patients to unnecessary risks. Discussing these issues with a homeopathic physician can help determine the best course of action when faced with difficult decisions.

With all that said, it must be acknowledged that it is not unusual for patients who seek help from outside the medical mainstream to find themselves conflicted over decisions regarding their health care. Patients may find that the advice they receive from their homeopathic doctors can diverge from their conventional doctors' advice. They may understandably feel caught in the middle.

It is not realistic to expect to be able to thoroughly discuss the advantages and disadvantages of allopathic testing and treatment versus homeopathic treatment with most allopathic doctors. Mainstream medicine's paternalistic attitude toward all perceived outside interference, especially any involvement having to do with holistic therapies, does nothing to help such situations. Given orthodoxy's general closed-mindedness, it is often left to the homeopathic physician to help patients navigate the conventional medical system. This basic truth cannot be denied, and is less than ideal, but the fault falls squarely at the doorstep of orthodox medicine. It is preferable, therefore, for patients to seek advice from medical personnel who are willing to discuss *all* of their concerns and therapeutic options.

Given this unfortunate state of affairs, it is important that patients understand that it is their right to choose and their right to refuse. It is their right to ask questions and their right to say, "no." Although mainstream medicine gives lip service to such rights, many doctors act offended when they perceive that their authority is being challenged—and sometimes when patients just dare to ask too many questions. Patient autonomy should be sacrosanct. As far as I am concerned, basic principles of medical freedom should be elevated to universal human rights. Of course, there are rare exceptions that need to be thoughtfully considered, as in the cases of children and certain adults who are incapable of making decisions for themselves.

The flip side of the patient autonomy issue is patient responsibility. If we wish to preserve our medical freedoms we also need to accept responsibility for our choices and decisions. The truth is that there are never any guarantees when it comes to health care outcomes, no matter how slam dunk a therapy or procedure is purported to be. Medicine surely plays a role in creating such unrealistic expectations. The image of scientific certainty that it projects is largely to blame. Ultimately, the general public needs to be less gullible about medical propaganda, which is eagerly propagated by the medical establishment and the media. The general public needs to take its role in the health care relationship more seriously. The best way to do that is through self-education.

Given the minefield created by medical overreach, patients need to develop strategies that they can employ when dealing with uncooperative or paternalistic medical personnel. I advise my patients never to burn their bridges, no matter how difficult a physician's behavior may become. The truth is that most people eventually need the medical system, so it is best to maintain diplomatic relations.

There is good reason why many patients do not fully disclose their involvement with holistic therapies to their doctors; they rightly fear that that information will be met with disapproval. When faced with a physician who is being difficult or disrespectful, it is preferable to say, "thank you doctor," before turning around and walking out the door. It is usually possible to find another doctor who will be more receptive. Similarly, patients can accept prescriptions but wait to fill them until they have had adequate time to discuss their situations with other qualified practitioners whom they trust. If a person feels too intimidated to ask his or her doctor questions, it can be helpful to bring along another family member or friend who is willing to ask those questions.

We hear a great deal from medicine about the need to gain patient compliance. This type of language is indicative of a larger need to educate mainstream medicine about patient rights. Patient compliance is a paternalistic concept. Mutual cooperation is the preferred ideal. It is ideal for patients to work with conventional physicians who are willing to listen to their concerns, respect their choices, and are interested in maintaining collegial relationships with their holistic and homeopathic practitioners.

The bottom line is that each individual is his or her own best advocate. The medical system often has its own agendas that don't necessarily align with patients' needs. It is imperative, therefore, for patients to learn to use the system to their advantage, to exercise their right of choice, and to take responsibility for their decisions in order to see to it that they get the care that they need and deserve. Until the day comes when orthodox and homeopathic medical camps learn to work together, the burden falls to patients to ensure that their voices are heard. This is one of the reasons why I have written this book.

Epigraphs & Notes

Foreword

Epigraph: James Tyler Kent, MD, *New Remedies, Clinical Cases, Lesser Writings, Aphorisms and Precepts*, Ehrhart and Karl, Chicago, 1926, *Series in Degrees*, pp. 356-360.

Chapter 1

Epigraph: E. A. Farrington, MD, *Therapeutic Pointers and Lesser Writings with Some Clinical Cases*, Salzer & Co, Calcutta, 1936, p. 13.

Epigraph: Margery Blackie, MD, *The Patient, Not the Cure: The Challenge of Homeopathy*, Macdonald and Jane's, London, 1976, p. 11.

1. Yasseri T., Spoerri A., Graham M., and Kertész J., *The most controversial topics in Wikipedia: A multilingual and geographical analysis*. In: Fichman P., Hara N., editors, Global Wikipedia: International and cross-cultural issues in online collaboration. Scarecrow Press (2014).

2. E. A. Farrington, MD, *Therapeutic Pointers and Lesser Writings with Some Clinical Cases*, Salzer & Co, Calcutta, 1936, p. 10.

3. Samuel Hahnemann, MD, *Organon Der Rationellen Heilkunde*, Arnoldischen Buchhandlung, 1810. (The first English translation of this first edition was published in 1913: Samuel Hahnemann. *The Organon of the Rational Art of Healing* translated by Charles E Wheeler, JM Dent & EP Dutton.)

4. Samuel Hahnemann, MD, *Organon of the Medical Art*, Edited and annotated by Wenda Brewster O'Reilly, Adapted from the sixth edition of the *Organon*, 1842, Redmond, Washington: Birdcage Books, 1996, p. 65.

5. Samuel Hahnemann, MD, *Organon of the Medical Art*, Edited and annotated by Wenda Brewster O'Reilly, Adapted from the sixth edition of the *Organon*, 1842, Redmond, Washington: Birdcage Books, 1996, p. 68.

6. Samuel Hahnemann, MD, *Organon of the Medical Art*, Edited and annotated by Wenda Brewster O'Reilly, Adapted from the sixth edition of the *Organon*, 1842, Redmond, Washington: Birdcage Books, 1996, p. 70.

7. Wilhelm Ameke, MD, *History of Homœopathy: Its Origins; Its Conflicts*, E. Gould & Son, London, 1883, p. 116.

Chapter 2

Epigraph: Stuart N. Close, MD, *The Genius of Homeopathy: Lectures and Essays on Homeopathic Philosophy*, Boericke & Tafel, Philadelphia, 1924, p. 53.

8. The first remedy to suspect in a case of right-sided pneumonia with a dry cough made worse by motion is *Bryonia alba*. One must consider this remedy in all cases where symptoms are aggravated by motion.

9. Suspect the remedy, *Antimonium tartaricum*, in pneumonia with a rattling cough. Although the lungs seem to be filled with fluid, the patient is unable to expectorate and coughs up little mucus. As is always the case, there may be other remedies with similar symptom profiles. More details regarding the particular case of pneumonia would be required to choose from among them.

Chapter 3

Epigraph: Garth Boericke, MD, *A Compend of the Principles of Homeopathy for Students in Medicine*, Boericke & Tafel, 1929, Philadelphia, p. 18.

10. The remedy that solved this case was *Drosera rotundifolia*. It can be useful in cases of violent paroxysmal coughing. The cough can be associated with muscle cramping and may be so severe as to induce nosebleeds. This is the type of cough often seen in croup and whooping cough.

11. The remedy indicated in this case was *Coccus cacti*. It is interesting to note that this remedy is made from a tiny little bug known to infest cactus plants. The symptoms of this remedy can be likened to having one of these little critters lodged in the larynx, producing copious amounts of ropey mucus and causing one to cough incessantly.

12. James responded nicely to *Mercurius vivus* (also known as *Mercurius solubilis*), which is a remedy that can work for a broad spectrum of health problems. It can be helpful for sore throats, tonsillitis, and mononucleosis. Like the mercury in a thermometer, persons who need *Mercurius* often complain of feeling sensitive to slight variations in the ambient temperature.

13. I will never forget this case and how quickly it responded to the remedy, *Lachesis muta*. This remedy made from the venom of the South American bushmaster snake was first introduced to the *materia medica* by the famous homeopath, Constantine Hering, MD. The very same specimen from which Hering extracted the venom is preserved today in a jar at the Academy of Natural Sciences at Drexel University. The specimen was originally held by the Philadelphia Medical College of Homeopathy, which Hering helped found in 1848. The college eventually became Hahnemann Hospital and was subsequently absorbed into the Drexel University College of Medicine.

14. This case responded nicely to *Psorinum*, another remedy brought to us courtesy of Dr. Hering. It is an example of what homeopaths call a nosode, a remedy made from a disease product. In order to make the nosode, Hering collected the discharge from skin pustules of a person presumably infected by the scabies mite.

15. *Kreosotum* is made from creosote, which is a preparation made from distilled beechwood tar. The primary focus of this remedy is the mucus membranes, which become inflamed and irritated with a tendency to bleed. It is useful for a wide array of female health problems.

16. *Phosphorus* is a commonly indicated polychrest remedy. A polychrest is a remedy with broad applicability toward a variety of mental, emotional, and physical health issues. Polychrests can often be recognized by their general characteristics. Some of the general features of *Phosphorus* include strong thirst for cold drinks, desire for spicy foods, chocolate, and ice cream, fear of thunderstorms, and an optimistic, friendly, sympathetic disposition.

17. *Spongia tosta* is a remedy made from the sea sponge found in the Mediterranean Sea. Like a sponge out of water, one of the defining features of *Spongia* symptomatology is dryness. It is useful for respiratory problems, endocrine disorders, and even cardiac conditions. Dry throat, dry cough, croup, laryngitis, and asthma are common indications for *Spongia*.

18. St. John's Wort is an herb familiar to many. In its homeopathic form, it is called *Hypericum perforatum*. It is especially helpful for puncture wounds and injuries that involve nerve-rich parts of the body such as the fingertips, tailbone, and eyeball. *Hypericum* is routinely used to speed recovery after dental procedures that involve anesthetic injections designed to deaden the nerves.

19. The remedy needed here was *Thuja occidentalis*. It is derived from an evergreen tree called the American arborvitae, which translates into "tree of life." As a homeopathic remedy, it is famous for its ability to treat warts. Someday when it is finally recognized as the remarkable healing agent that it truly is, *Thuja* will make a world of difference for the many thousands of individuals who suffer from the chronic consequences of adverse vaccine reactions.

20. *Natrum muriaticum* is another famous homeopathic polychrest with broad applicability. Amazingly, it is derived from simple rock salt, a form of sodium chloride. To think that such an ordinary substance can heal so deeply is a revelation to all homeopaths. People who need this remedy can be recognized by their preference for salt, chocolate, and starchy foods, in addition to their high degree

of emotional independence. They do not like to talk about personal issues.

21. Some homeopathic remedies are derived from animal poisons such as snake venoms. Other remedies are made from the entire poisonous animal, as in this case. *Tarentula hispanica* is a preparation made from the whole spider, a tarantula found in regions of Spain and Italy. People who respond to this remedy are quick and agile, with restless bodies and busy minds. They can be very sensitive to music and color.

22. *Carcinosinum* is one of the most improbable yet indispensible healing agents that one can possibly imagine. Another example of a nosode, this remedy is made from a discharge obtained from breast cancer tissue. It is a very broad and deep acting remedy, one that is particularly valuable in this modern age in which cancer is so prevalent.

Chapter 4

Epigraph: George Royal, MD, *A Handy Book of Reference for Students and General Practitioners of Homœopathy*, Boericke & Tafel, Philadelphia, 1930, p. 20.

Epigraph: Willis A. Dewey, MD, *Essentials of Homœopathic Materia Medica and Homœopathic Pharmacy Being a Quiz Compend*, Boericke & Tafel, Philadelphia, 1908, p. 15.

Epigraph: George Royal, MD, *A Handy Book of Reference for Students and General Practitioners of Homœopathy*, Boericke & Tafel, Philadelphia, 1930, p. 31.

23. Julian Winston, *The Heritage of Homœopathic Literature: An Abbreviated Bibliography and Commentary*, Great Auk Publishing, Tawa, New Zealand, 2001, p. xi.

24. William Boericke, MD, *Pocket Manual of Homœopathic Materia Medica*, Boericke and Runyon, Philadelphia, 1901.

25. James Tyler Kent, MD, *Lectures on Homeopathic Materia Medica*, Boericke & Tafel, Philadelphia, 1905.

26. George Vithoulkas, *Essence of Materia Medica*, Gazelle Distribution Trade, 2008.
27. Rajan Sankaran, MD, *The Spirit of Homeopathy*, Homœopathic Medical Publishers, Bombay, 1992.
28. Rajan Sankaran, MD, *The Soul of Remedies*, Homeopathic Medical Publishers, Bombay, 1997, p. 121. (The remedy, *Lyssinum*, is actually made from the saliva of a rabid dog and was first proven by Constantine Hering, MD in 1833.)
29. James Tyler Kent, MD, *A Repertory of Homœopathic Materia Medica*, Examiner Printing House, Lancaster, PA, 1900.
30. Based on these few details, *Belladonna* would be the best choice of remedy. In its natural plant form, the Deadly Nightshade is a powerful poison that causes circulatory disturbances. It causes pulsating sensations and pains, and rushing of blood to various parts of the body, thus causing those parts to turn bright red. In its homeopathic form, *Belladonna* is completely benign.
31. These modalities make *Bryonia alba* the most likely choice of remedy. The "keynote" or standout feature of *Bryonia* is that many of its symptoms are made worse from any kind of motion. It is commonly indicated for acute illnesses like coughs, flu, and viral illnesses, especially when movement aggravates the headache, cough, aches, and pains. It is also useful for any injury that is aggravated by motion. The person who needs *Bryonia* wishes to remain quiet and still.
32. *Rhus toxicodendron* is a remedy made from poison ivy. It can be conceptualized as the complementary opposite to *Bryonia*. While *Bryonia* symptoms are worse from motion, *Rhus tox* symptoms are ameliorated by motion. More specifically, *Rhus tox* symptoms are briefly worse upon initial motion, better from continued motion, and worse again from overuse. Think of the person with a bad back who feels pain and stiffness on rising from sitting, feels bet-

ter after "walking it off," and then aggravates the back again by overexerting.

Chapter 5

Epigraph: Herbert A. Roberts, MD, *Principles & Art of Cure by Homœopathy*, Health Science Press, Rustington, England, 1936, p. 94.

33. Wilhelm Ameke, MD, *History of Homœopathy: Its Origins; Its Conflicts*, E. Gould & Son, London, 1883, p. 330.

34. The most thorough discussion of the paradoxical phenomenon of similars, both in nature and homeopathy, is to be found in Dr. Steven Goldsmith's book: *The Healing Paradox: A Revolutionary Approach to Treating and Curing Physical and Mental Illness*, North Atlantic Books, Berkeley, California, 2013.

35. For an in-depth explanation of the Arndt-Schulz principle and its relationship to homeopathy, I recommend: *Arndt Schulz Law and its Applications*, Rajneesh Kumar Sharma, MD (Hom), February 9, 2011. http://www.homeopathyworldcommunity.com/profiles/blogs/arndt-schultz-law-and-its

36. Chester M. Southam, Focusing on the Dose-Response in the Low-Dose Zone, International Dose-Response Society, UMassAmherst, Department of Public Health, Environmental Health Sciences. http://dose-response.org/chester-m-southam/

37. Davenas E, Beauvais F, Amara J, et al. (June 1988). *Human basophil degranulation triggered by very dilute antiserum against IgE*. Nature 333 (6176): 816-8.

38. Wynn Free with Jacques Benveniste, MD, *Digital Biology and the Memory of Water*, The Spirit of Maat, Vol 3 No 5. http://www.spiritofmaat.com/archive/dec3/bveniste.htm

39. Newsmaker interview: *Luc Montagnier, French Nobelist Escapes 'Intellectual Terror' to Pursue Radical Ideas in China*. Science, 24 December 2010; 330, 1732.

40. Newsmaker interview: *Luc Montagnier, French Nobelist Escapes 'Intellectual Terror' to Pursue Radical Ideas in China*. Science, 24 December 2010; 330, 1732.

41. Wikipedia Page: Rupert Sheldrake, https://en.wikipedia.org/wiki/Rupert_Sheldrake

42. Chikramane, Prashant Satish et al. *Extreme homeopathic dilutions retain starting materials: A nanoparticulate perspective.* Homeopathy, Volume 99, Issue 4, 231-242. http://www.homeopathyjournal.net/article/S1475-4916(10)00054-8/abstract?cc=y=

43. Bell IR, Koithan M. *A model for homeopathic remedy effects: low dose nanoparticles, allostatic cross-adaptation, and time-dependent sensitization in a complex adaptive system.* BMC Complementary and Alternative Medicine. 2012; 12:191. doi:10.1186/1472-6882-12-191. http://bmccomplementalternmed.biomedcentral.com/articles/10.1186/1472-6882-12-191

44. *Homeopathic Basic Science Research*, Foundation for PIHMA, Research and Education. http://pihma-fpre.org/homeopathic-basic-science-research

45. *Natrum muriaticum*, homeopathic sodium chloride, is the same remedy that was used for the young girl in Chapter 3 (page 25) who manifested her stress through her skin in the form of molluscum contagiosum. Both she and this man with hives display a strong tendency to internalize their emotions.

46. This is a case of *Sepia officinalis*, which was described in detail in the previous chapter. In this particular case, it is reasonable to think that the depression may have originated with the onset of this young girl's menses. Compare this case with the *materia medica* description in Chapter 4 (page 59).

47. *Colocynthis*, also known as the Bitter Cucumber, can be useful for menstrual cramps, intestinal cramps, or any type of cramp associated with strong feelings of anger or indignation. The symptoms of

this remedy are ameliorated by warmth, hard pressure, and bending double or curling up into a ball.

48. Interestingly, *Lachesis muta* is the same remedy that miraculously resolved the case of enormously swollen tonsils in Chapter 3 (page 25). The psychological profile of the person who needs *Lachesis* often includes jealousy (sometimes to the point of paranoia), possessiveness, a need to control others, loquaciousness, and its famous fear of snakes. Many such individuals will not admit to their fear of snakes. They tend, instead, to say that they "don't like" snakes.

49. Larry Malerba, DO, *Green Medicine: Challenging the Assumptions of Conventional Health Care*, North Atlantic Books, Berkeley, California, 2010.

50. Samuel Hahnemann, MD, *Organon of the Medical Art*, Edited and annotated by Wenda Brewster O'Reilly, Adapted from the sixth edition of the *Organon*, 1842, Redmond, Washington: Birdcage Books, 1996, p. 68.

51. Larry Malerba, DO, *Metaphysics & Medicine: Restoring Freedom of Thought to the Art and Science of Healing*, Maverick Press, New York, 2014.

Chapter 6

Epigraph: Stuart N. Close, MD, *The Genius of Homeopathy: Lectures and Essays on Homeopathic Philosophy*, Boericke & Tafel, Philadelphia, 1924, p. 62.

Epigraph: Herbert A. Roberts, MD, *Principles & Art of Cure by Homœopathy*, Health Science Press, Rustington, England, 1936, pp. 37-38.

52. Helen Thomson, *Study of Holocaust survivors finds trauma passed on to children's genes*, www.theguardian.com, August 21, 2015. http://www.theguardian.com/science/2015/aug/21/study-of-holocaust-survivors-finds-trauma-passed-on-to-childrens-genes

53. *Opium* is a substance that can induce dream-like states of unreality, not unlike this mother who had a terror-induced out-of-body

experience. Opium in its crude form can induce distortions of consciousness, states of sleepiness with heavy dreaming, shallow breathing, and constipation. Homeopathic *Opium*, therefore, is indicated for people who complain of similar symptoms.

54. Herbert A. Roberts, MD, *Principles & Art of Cure by Homœopathy*, Health Science Press, Rustington, England, 1936, p. 37.

55. This is the symptom picture of *Ignatia amara*, the most commonly indicated remedy for acute states of grief. The emotions are intense, unpredictable, and volatile. The person alternates between trying to control and losing control of strong feelings of grief and sadness, with sudden bouts of sobbing and crying. In the old homeopathic books, this unique emotional state was often characterized as "hysteria."

56. *Aurum metallicum* is a homeopathic remedy prepared from the precious metal, gold. It is known for its bleak states of dark depression that can be triggered by grief or a feeling of having failed to meet one's own expectations in life. I have seen this remedy pull many people out of serious states of depression, oftentimes giving them a sense of purpose in life that had been previously missing.

57. In this case, grief manifests in such a way as to make it look more like the person is suffering from fatigue or depression. *Phosphoricum acidum* is the ideal remedy for such situations. While there may be a history of grief or loss in the person's life, the main complaint is more likely to be apathy, lack of motivation, fatigue, and a tendency to sleep late in the mornings and to while away the hours like a couch potato.

58. Rupert Sheldrake, *The Science Delusion: Freeing the Spirit of Enquiry* (Later published as *Science Set Free*) Coronet, Hodder & Stoughton Ltd, London, 2012, pp. 99-100.

59. *Veratrum album* is a remedy derived from a flowering plant called the white hellebore. Its broad scope of action makes it useful in treating everything from diarrhea and vomiting to ADHD and

bipolar disorder. As noted, the person who needs *Veratrum* is often quite cold but yet craves ice-cold food and drink. Another peculiar clue indicating this remedy is the craving for salty and sour foods, especially sour fruits.

60. The homeopathic literature famously refers to *Nux vomica* as the main remedy for "debauchery." Digestive derangement is a common consequence of overindulgence in culinary pleasures. The combination of nausea, cramping, chilliness, and irritability is a strong indicator for *Nux vomica*, which is one of the great polychrest remedies. Its scope includes the aftermath of all kinds of excesses, including the abuse of food, alcohol, stimulants like coffee, prescription drugs, and recreational drugs. *Nux vomica* is the mainstay of any homeopathic detox program.

61. *Sulphur* is a commonly indicated "constitutional" remedy. Typical *Sulphur* persons are warm-blooded, love hot spicy foods, tend to be sloppy and disorganized, and have a know-it-all attitude that causes them to engage in debate with others. When the *Sulphur* type person gets sick, he or she may complain of burning pains and sensations. There is also a specific pattern to the diarrhea attacks, which tend to wake the person from sleep in the early morning, especially around 5am.

Chapter 7

Epigraph: James Tyler Kent, MD, *Lectures on Homœopathic Philosophy*, Ehrhart & Karl, Chicago, Memorial Edition, 1919 (Copyrighted 1900), p. 40.

62. Carroll Dunham, MD, *The Science of Therapeutics*, Boericke & Tafel, Philadelphia, 1877, p. 19.

63. *Arsenicum album* is a remedy made from arsenic. In its crude form, it is toxic. In homeopathic dilution, it is harmless. The *Arsenicum* patient is neat, tidy, and persnickety, with a tendency toward anxiety about personal security. Financial insecurity and physical illness represent the two main threats to this type of patient. It is one

of the main remedies for chronic anxiety about health. The person is often impeccably dressed and has a tendency to get cold easily. There is usually a preference for warm drinks.

64. *Calcarea carbonica*, along with *Sulphur* and *Lycopodium clavatum*, completes the famous triad of homeopathic constitutional polychrests. It is derived from the calcium carbonate obtained from an oyster shell. *Calcarea* persons have endomorphic body types, are generally chilly, prefer a traditional farm-based diet that includes eggs, meat, and potatoes, and are temperamentally slow, steady, practical, and responsible. *Calcarea* types have a distinct tendency to worry and are prone to fears regarding their capacity to function independently in the world. Their worst nightmare would be to be confined to a wheelchair or a nursing home.

65. *Mancinella venenata* is a plant-based remedy. Although it is a less commonly prescribed remedy, it nevertheless has a very specific indication. It is suited to persons who are obsessed about evil or demonic forces. They fear evil, supernatural forces, and possession by the devil. The trend that began with the movie, *The Exorcist*, continues to this day. The growing legion of individuals traumatized by so many spiritually twisted horror movies would do well to consult a homeopath for their psychic pain and suffering. A remedy like *Mancinella* could change their lives.

66. Samuel Hahnemann, MD, *Organon of the Art of Healing*, Translated from the fifth German edition by C. Wesselhoft, MD, Boericke & Tafel, Philadelphia, 1881, p. 174.

Chapter 8

Epigraph: James Tyler Kent, MD, *Lectures on Homœopathic Philosophy*, Ehrhart & Karl, Chicago, Memorial Edition, 1919 (Copyrighted 1900), p. 28.

Epigraph: Rajan Sankaran, MD, *The Spirit of Homeopathy*, Homœopathic Medical Publishers, Bombay, 1992, p. 50.

67. Dr. André Saine, D.C., N.D., F.C.A.H., *Hering's Law: Law, Rule or Dogma?* Presented at the Second Annual Session of the Homeopathic Academy of Naturopathic Physicians in Seattle, Washington, April 16-17, 1988.
http://www.homeopathy.ca/articles_det12.shtml

68. Larry Malerba, DO, *Green Medicine: Challenging the Assumptions of Conventional Health Care*, North Atlantic Books, Berkeley, California, 2010.

69. If you refer back to Chapter 4 (page 49) and the case in Chapter 5 (page 63), it should be clear that this is another example of a patient who needs *Sepia officinalis*. In this case, symptomatology has been triggered by menopause. Sadly, this type of hormonal depression can sometimes drive a wedge between two previously happily married persons. Fortunately, I have seen homeopathy correct such hormonal imbalances and, in the process, save more than a few marriages.

70. *Kali bichromicum* is made from potassium bichromate. It is known for the keynote symptom of tenacious mucus that can be hard to expectorate from the respiratory passages. It is also known to fit a pattern of alternating symptoms whereby one set of symptoms emerges as another set of symptoms recedes. Most commonly, respiratory symptoms alternate with arthritic or gastrointestinal symptoms. We see in this case how the long forgotten sciatica reemerges as the sinus problems resolve.

71. Samuel Hahnemann, MD, *Organon of the Medical Art*, Edited and annotated by Wenda Brewster O'Reilly, Adapted from the sixth edition of the *Organon*, 1842, Redmond, Washington: Birdcage Books, 1996, p. 64.

Chapter 9

Epigraph: Margery Blackie, MD, *The Patient, Not the Cure: The Challenge of Homeopathy*, Macdonald and Jane's, London, 1976, p. 167.

Epigraph: Wilhelm Ameke, MD, *History of Homœopathy: Its Origins; Its Conflicts*, E. Gould & Son, London, 1883, p. iii.

72. See Chapter 14, Larry Malerba, DO, *Metaphysics & Medicine: Restoring Freedom of Thought to the Art and Science of Healing*, Maverick Press, New York, 2014.

73. British Homeopathic Association, *The evidence for homeopathy*, www.britishhomeopathic.org. http://www.britishhomeopathic.org/evidence/the-evidence-for-homeopathy/.
Also: https://www.hri-research.org/resources/homeopathy-faqs/there-is-no-scientific-evidence-homeopathy-works/

74. El Dib RP, Atallah AN, Andriolo RB (2007). *Mapping the Cochrane evidence for decision making in health care.* Journal of Evaluation in Clinical Practice; 13:689-692. http://onlinelibrary.wiley.com/doi/10.1111/j.1365-2753.2007.00886.x/abstract

75. Thomas Kuhn, *The Structure of Scientific Revolutions*, University of Chicago Press, 1962.

76. Here again, we have a scenario that warrants a prescription of *Natrum muriaticum*. In this case, it is depicted in a way that might happen during an actual patient visit. This patient doesn't just come right out and say, "I have grief-induced arthritis." As with most cases, it must be deduced from the information presented. I have seen a number of cases of grief-induced rheumatoid arthritis completely resolved by this remedy. Two additional features of *Natrum muriaticum* include a tendency to develop mouth sores from emotional stress and/or exposure to sun, and a modality that involves aggravation of symptoms around 10am.

77. You may recall from Chapter 4 (page 49) that *Rhus toxicodendron* symptoms are ameliorated from continued motion. It is a great remedy for arthritic complaints and injuries, especially injuries that result in long term stiffness. Knowing that *Rhus tox* is made from poison ivy, it should come as no surprise that it is also beneficial in conditions that involve blistering, such as herpes, chicken pox, and shingles.

Chapter 10

Epigraph: James Tyler Kent, MD, *Lectures on Homœopathic Philosophy*, Ehrhart & Karl, Chicago, Memorial Edition, 1919 (Copyrighted 1900), p. 50.

Epigraph: Elizabeth Danciger, *Homeopathy: From Alchemy to Medicine*, Healing Arts Press, Rochester, Vermont, 1987, pp. 2-3.

78. Charles J. Hempel, MD, *The Science of Homœopathy*, Boericke & Tafel, Philadelphia, 1874, p. vii.

Appendix

79. Larry Malerba, DO, *Homeopathic Arnica to the Rescue*, Huffington Post, 2011. http://www.huffingtonpost.com/larry-malerba/homeopathic-arnica_b_1081164.html

About the Author

Larry Malerba, DO, DHt is a classical homeopath, osteopathic physician, and author whose mission is to build bridges between holistic healing, conventional medicine, and spirituality. Dr. Malerba is board certified in Homeotherapeutics and past president of the Homeopathic Medical Society of the State of New York.

Books by Dr. Malerba:

- Green Medicine: Challenging the Assumptions of Conventional Health Care

- Metaphysics & Medicine: Restoring Freedom of Thought to the Art and Science of Healing

Facebook: facebook.com/LarryMalerba
Twitter: twitter.com/docmalerba
Minds: minds.com/DocMalerba
SpiritScienceHealing.com

www.ingramcontent.com/pod-product-compliance
Lightning Source LLC
Chambersburg PA
CBHW020250030426
42336CB00010B/695